CHRONIC PAIN

Reflex Sympathetic Dystrophy
Prevention and Management

Hooshang Hooshmand, M.D.

CRC Press
Boca Raton   Ann Arbor   London   Tokyo

Library of Congress Cataloging-in-Publication Data

Hooshmand, H. (Hooshang)
    Chronic pain: reflex sympathetic dystrophy. Prevention and management / H. Hooshmand.
       p. cm.
    Includes bibliographical references and index.
    ISBN 0-8493-8667-5
    1. Reflex sympathetic dystrophy. 2. Intractable pain. I. Title.
    [DNLM: 1. Chronic Disease. 2. Pain. 3. Reflex Sympathetic Dystrophy—diagnosis. 4. Reflex Sympa-
thetic Dystrophy—etiology. 5. Reflex Sympathetic Dystrophy—therapy. 6. Sympathetic Nervous System—
physiopathology. WL 600 H789c 1993]
    RC422.R43H66 1993
    616′.0472—dc20
    DNLM/DLC
    for Library of Congress   92-48334
                                                                CIP

International Standard Book Number 0-8493-8667-5

Library of Congress Card Number 92-48334
Printed in the United States   3 4 5 6 7 8 9 0
Printed on acid-free paper

ACKNOWLEDGMENT

This work is dedicated to J. J. Bonica, M.D., who has devoted his life to helping physicians learn more about pain.

ABOUT THE AUTHOR

Hooshang Hooshmand, M.D. practices intractable neurology in Vero Beach, Florida: managing intractable pain, intractable epilepsy, and intractable multiple sclerosis. He had his training in neurosurgery and neurology in the Mayo Clinic. He was professor of neurology at the Medical College of Virginia for eight years. He has published over 80 scientific papers and 6 chapters of books on the subject of neurolgy.

He is the recipient of research awards by the American Congress of Neurosurgery as well as the AMA.

His pioneering works in diagnosis and management of electrical injuries, management of neurosyphilis, application of clonazepam in intractable seizures, and application of ACTH in treatment of chronic pain are some of his original contributions.

His interest in the subject of complex chronic pain of RSD dates back to his experience in RSD and sympathectomy as early as his neurosurgery training in the Mayo Clinic 30 years ago. He is a strong believer in preventive medicine and avoidance of surgery.

He was the teacher of the year in 1971, 1972, and 1973 at the Medical College of Virginia. His passion for teaching is reflected in his writings — including this book.

TABLE OF CONTENTS

DETAILED CONTENTS

TABLE OF FIGURES

LIST OF TABLES

ACRONYMS

ACTH	Adrenocorticotropic hormone
AIDS	Aquired immune deficiency syndrome
BAEP	Brain stem auditory evoked potentials
BEP	Brain-evoked potentials
BER	Brain stem-evoked response
BZ	Benzodiazepine
CCK	Cholecystokinine
CCP	Complex chronic pain
CSF	Cerebrospinal fluid
CNS	Central nervous system
DEEG	Depth EEG
DNA	Deoxyribonucleic acid
EEG	Electroencephalography
EM	Electromicroscopy
EMG	Electromyography
EMR	Electromagnetic resonance imaging
EP	Evoked potentials
EMEG	Electromagnetic encephalography
ENG	Electronystagmography
FAS	Fetal alcohol syndrome
LH	Luteinizing hormone
MEG	Magnetic encephalography
MR	Magnetic resonance
MRI	Magnetic resonance imaging
MRS	Magnetic resonance spectrometry
MSA	Multiple system atrophy
PAF	Pure, primary autonomic failure
PCA	Patient-controlled analgesia
PET	Positron emission tomography
PNS	Peripheral nervous system
POMC	Proopiomelanocortin
RNA	Ribonucleic acid
RSD	Reflex sympathetic dysfunction; Reflex sympathetic dystrophy
SEP	Somatosensory evoked potentials
SER	Sensory-evoked response
SIA	Stress-induced analgesia
SIF	Small intensity fluorescent (cells)
SIP	Stress-induced pain
SMP	Sympathetically mediated pain
SNS	Sympathetic nervous system
SSEP	Somatosensory evoked potentials
TBM	Topographic brain mapping
TMJ	Temporomandibular joint disease
TNS	Transcutaneous nerve stimulator
TPI	Trigger point injection
WDR	Wide dynamic range
VEP	Visual-evoked potentials
VER	Visual-evoked response
XMT	Cross-modality transmission (of pain)

PREFACE

Pain is the common thread that weaves all the medical disciplines — medicine, dentistry, osteopathy, or chiropractic — together.

Pain is multidimensional (Figure 1a). In its most common form, **acute pain**, it is a simple somatic defense of transient nature. Acute pain is by and large harmless and benign. Cancer is the main exception by causing relentless destruction and longstanding repetitive acute pain.

Chronic pain has a tendency to persist long after the occurrence of the original noxious injury. In and of itself chronic pain need not be miserable or intractable. Older people often wake up with some chronic aches and pain.

When chronic pain becomes complicated, it becomes hard to control. **Complex chronic pain** (CCP) adversely stimlates multiple areas of the nervous system. This multidimensional aspect of chronic pain taxes the patience of the clinician.

The temporal factor (chronicity) is not enough to qualify the pain as complex (CCP). Chronic pain complicated by one or more of the following factors passes for CCP:

1. Involvement of the **sympathetic system** and resultant abnormal vicious circle of **vasoconstriction, inactivity**, and perpetuation of pain due to **reflex sympathetic dysfunction** (RSD).

$$\text{Chronic pain (CP)} + \text{RSD} = \text{CCP}$$

2. **Depression** in the form of emotional exhaustion and insomnia — usually due to longstanding use of narcotics or benzodiazepines and at times due to social and financial difficulties — can change the pain to CCP.

$$\text{CP} + \text{Depression} = \text{CCP}$$

3. **Stress-induced pain** (SIP) due to **distress** of inactivity or other pathologic stressful factors is the opposite of stress (eustress)-induced analgesia (SIA).
   Distress and Eustress are discussed in detail in this book (see Chapter 4).

$$\text{CP} + \text{SIP} = \text{CCP}$$

4. Aggravation of CP with permanent central or peripheral nerve damage and scar is enough to cause CCP. A neuroma (e.g., phantom pain), a scar in the brain stem or thalamus, or a scar in a peripheral nerve trunk (e.g., ephaptic causalgia or nerve contusion) changes CP to CCP.

$$\text{CP} + \text{neuroma or nerve contusion} = \text{CCP}$$

Complex chronic pain in contrast with acute or chronic pain mainly stimulates the **limbic system** through the paleospinothalamic tract, discussed in detail in this book. The stimulation results in panic, depression, and low threshold for pain.

Reflex sympathetic dysfunction is a form of CCP that mainly stimulates the limbic system and causes highly **emotional hyperpathic pain** (Figure 21a).

RSD, the "pain that never stops", is not rare. The advent of thermography has helped us realize that RSD comprises between 10 and 20% of chronic pain patients. At any given time, chronic pain grounds one third of the workforce according to medical economists. These facts indicate that there are approximately 4 million disabled RSD patients in the United States.

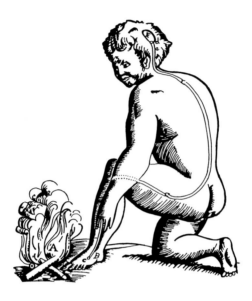

FIGURE 1. Drawing from a book entitled *L'Homme* by the famous philosopher René Descartes (C. Angot, Paris, 1664). The noxious stimulus (A) is transmitted to the body (B) through peripheral and central nervous systems (C, D, E, and F). After centuries of debate, it is clear that chronic pain (especially RSD) is perceived and modulated in all levels of peripheral nerves and tissues as well as central nervous system (C, D, E, and F). This theroy is still the best theory explaining the afferent portion of the sensory and motor arch of reflex sympathetic dystrophy.

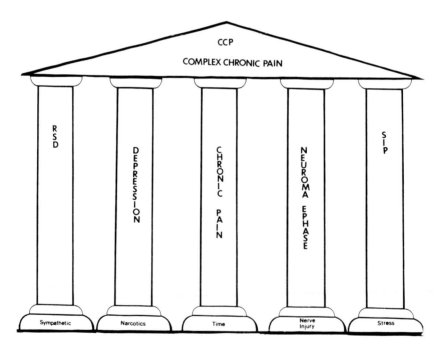

FIGURE 1a. Chronic complex pain. CCP, complex chronic pain; CP (chronic pain) + D (depression) = CCP: CP + RSD = CCP; CP + NI (nerve injury) = CCP; SIP, stress induced pain; RSD, reflex sympathetic dystrophy.

The RSD form of CCP is more disabling than other forms of chronic pain, and it is less forgiving to the victim. It is more difficult to help the victims of RSD to return to work and to a normal life — unless the disease is diagnosed early and treated properly. A well-performed study by Poplawski sponsored by the Canadian Office of Workers' Compensation revealed that **early diagnosis** is the paramount requirement for successful management of RSD.

RSD is seen by practically all disciplines of medicine: physiatrists, neurologists, anesthesiologists, neurosurgeons, and orthopedists see such patients practically on a daily basis — yet they rarely diagnose such patients in early stages. Late diagnosis guarantees failure of treatment.

Dermatologists frequently treat dermal manifestations of RSD (herpes zooster, etc).

Pediatricians treat children with RSD but usually do not recognize the link between **movement disorders** or joint pains after trauma, or, for that matter, **posttraumatic migraine** headaches, and RSD.

Internists frequently deal with RSD but call it "neuralgia" due to diabetic neuropathy, or misdiagnose it as "Raynaud's phenomenon",[476a] which obviously has nothing to do with RSD.

Dentists and oral surgeons call it "TMJ disease", which can be present independently or in combination with RSD.

Plastic and hand surgeons call it "soft tissue injuries" and try to treat it surgically with disastrous end results.

Podiatrists call it "neuroma" and "remove" the painful nerve endings with obvious aggravation of RSD.

Chiropractors find the cause in "curvatures" and "subluxations" of spine.

There is no limit to this list. Eventually these patients are referred to psychiatrists and are silenced with potent "zomby" type medications such as haloperidol. No wonder one-third of the workforce is out of commission with chronic pain. No wonder heart attack and suicide are two extreme end results of patients with injuries that had originally been diagnosed as a minor "myofascial injury": a garbage-can terminology that has practically no tangible scientific connotation.

Early diagnosis, extensive sympathetic nerve blocks, and **physiotherapy**, as well as proper treatment with **antidepressants**, are essential to prevent any need for surgery. Sympathectomy is useless in the long run and should be resorted to when the patient has a short life expectancy (less than 5 years).

RSD does not limit itself to the extremities. RSD can occur over the **head and face** with manifestation of severe **migraine vascular headache**. Early and proper diagnosis and treatment can spare these patients from years of suffering.

A simple injury to nerves, muscles, or ligaments in the cervical paraspinal region goes undiagnosed and mistreated for years. Eventually a secondary vascular headache due to RSD sets in. The patient is then diagnosed with "migraine" or "cluster" headache and treated with metisergide or barbiturates. After proper diagnosis, simple physiotherapy, traction, and trigger point injection in such patients provide a lot more relief.

This book tries to summarize the facts about the complex subject of RSD. It is written with the hope that it may help the clinician understand the nature of this form of complex chronic pain.

The present state-of-the-art of the diagnosis and management of headache leaves a lot to be desired. The symptoms are mistaken for the cause; hence, vague terminology such as "classic migraine", "common migraine", etc. are considered diagnostic entities. The treatment ignores the cause and tries to shut the patient up by the use of strong and dangerous drugs such as narcotics or metysergide. If the patient still dares to complain, then depressive drugs such as propranolol or addictive drugs such as barbiturates and BZ's are used to dope the patient.

A careful history taking and a careful examination of the patient's **cervical spine** not infrequently reveals the source and the nature of the **headache**, resulting in successful treatment with physiotherapy, traction, etc.

The leaders in the field of headache such as Moskowitz realize that SNS can affect the craniofacial region as easily as it affects the extremities. The same principles of diagnosis and management applied for RSD can successfully be applied for vascular headaches.

This book attempts to bring to the attention of the clinician the common misconceptions of pain: that calling a headache "muscle tension" vs. "vascular headache" does not specify the cause for the disease. That sympathectomy is not a cure. That ACTH is not a "steroid". That early diagnosis complemented with sympathetic nerve block and physiotherapy are essential for treatment of RSD.

Introduction

Chronic pain is being mismanaged universally. Impatient surgeons try unsuccessfully to excise the pain. Internists load the patient with narcotics and depressing tranquilizers. Chiropractors try to cure everything with their fingers. Acupuncturists shoot darts at the patients.

The inevitable failure in control of pain is compounded by the hostile attitude of the impatient healer. The victim suffers from magnified pain due to the side effects of "treatment". The physician considers the patient crazy and relegates the pain management to the psychiatrist who is not trained in the management of pain.

Even this late in the twentieth century, the patient has to cope with the nonsensical accusation that "it's all in your head" where every kind of pain obviously resides.

The most misunderstood and complex subject in medicine is the hyperpathic pain of *sympathetic dystrophy*. Understanding this self-perpetuating pain — which "never stops" — requires unbiased knowledge of physiology and pathology. Above all, it requires the open mind of a physician who can understand that there is no dicotomy between "psyche" and "soma", between "brain" and "mind", or between "true" and "imagined" pain.

In contrast to somesthetic pain, sympathetic pain terminates in the limbic system. It can be more severe than the pain of cancer. It can be fatal: heart attack or suicide is more common among these patients than the rest of the population. It causes tremor, blepharospasm, flexion deformity, vasoconstriction, and severe vascular migraine headache.

RSD is more common than previously assumed by clinicians. Trauma is not at the top of the list of its variety of etiologies. It may have its origin in the periphery: head, cervical spine, trunk, or extremities. It may just as well originate in CNS: spinal cord, brain stem, or cerebral hemispheres.

Invasive surgical treatments in the form of sympathectomy, tractotomy, arthrodesis, or stimulative procedures are apt to fail in the long run. Narcotics, alcohol, and almost all benzodiazepines only exacerbate the sympathetic pain.

The physician can substantially increase the rate of success in the control of this intractable pain by taking advantage of early diagnosis, aggressive physiotherapy, multiple sympathetic blocks, as well as epidural blocks and antidepressants.

The goal of this book is to review the present knowledge regarding the understanding, prevention, and management of the scourge of reflex sympathetic dystrophy.

History of Reflex Sympathetic Dysfunction

HISTORY

"It would be a great thing to understand pain
in all its meanings."

Peter M. Latham

Reflex sympathetic dystrophy (RSD) is the most unpleasant and uncomfortable form of chronic pain. It is the extreme prototype of disabling chronic pain.

Chronic pain is the type of pain that persists long after the original injury. Obviously, recurrent attacks of acute pain due to new and repetitive damages from cancer or recurrent heart attack cannot be considered chronic pain even though they may be of longstanding duration.

It is estimated that approximately 30% of the general population suffers from chronic pain. One third of these patients suffers from RSD.

The chronic pain of RSD is typified by a marked **emotional connotation**. It is invariably accompanied by **anxiety, phobia**, and neuropsychological disturbances in the form of **irritability, agitation**, and **depression**.

Historically, chronic pain has been the subject of clinical debate among physicans for a few centuries. Greek philosophers considered the brain as the site of pain perception. The first references to hyperpathic sympathetic type of pain appeared in the literature in the late 1700s by the famous British surgeon Potts. He first mentioned that trauma can be the source of **burning pain** and **atrophy** of the extremity.[57]

The first report of amputation for treatment of this type of pain was by Denmark in 1813.[350] Even though **amputation** seems to be a drastic and extreme form of treatment for RSD, even at the present time surgeons are performing amputation for RSD accompanied by osteoporotic fractures.

Needless to say, no RSD patient should undergo amputation. Even multiple fractures in small bones of the foot can be corrected without surgery. Proper physiotherapy, weight-bearing, sympathetic blocks, etc., will always save the extremity from being amputated. However, amputation is done because of lack of understanding regarding the nature of RSD. It is done when all other measures have failed and especially because of the fact that only a small percentage of RSD patients are diagnosed in the early stages of the disease. By the time the disease becomes advanced, the pathology takes a rapidly accelerating downhill course that

TABLE 1
History

Year	Author	Contribution
1700	Potts	Burning pain and atrophy in injured extremity
1813	Denmark	Amputation for treatment of pain
1853	Bernard	Role of sympathetic system in temperature control
1878	Bernard	Role of sympathetic system in sustaining the balance of internal environment (Mileu Interne)
1864	S. Weir Mitchell	Erythromelalgia
1867	S. Weir Mitchell	Causalgia
1882	Volkmann	Posttraumatic bone rarefaction: "acute atrophy of bone"
1898	Destot	Singular osteoporosis due to longstanding sprained ankle
1900	Sudek	Atrophy and bone rarefaction secondary to nerve damage
1901	Santorio	Thermoscope
1908	Bier	The first regional block
1916	Leriche	Sympathectomy
1923	Orbeli	Antifatigue effect of sympathetic nerves (Orbeli effect)
1926	Leriche	Sympathetic nerve roots dysfunction as cause of pain
1926	Barré	Barré-Lieou syndrome, cervical pathology involving sympathetic nerves surrounding vertebral arteries causing vertigo, blurred vision, and pain in the arms
1928	Lieou	Sympathetic involvement in cervical spine pathology (Barré-Lieou syndrome)
1929	Zur Verth	Peripheral acute trophoneurosis
1931	Morton and Scott	Traumatic angiospasm
1932	Hisey	Brain as an endocrine gland (controlling ovulation)
1933	Fontaine and Herrmann	Posttraumatic osteoporosis and bone rarefaction
1934	Lehman	Traumatic vasospasm
1937	DeTakats	Reflex dystrophy
1940	Homans	Minor causalgia (in contrast to Mitchell's major causalgia)
1940	Ray and Wolff	Trigeminal nerve role in cranial vascular headache
1943	Livingston	Vicious circle of inactivity and pain resulting in RSD
1947	Steinbrocker	1. Reflex neurovascular dystrophy 2. Shoulder-hand syndrome with atrophy of hand as a common form of RSD
1947	Evans	The syndrome of reflex sympathetic dystrophy (RSDS)
1947	Nathan	Multiple level input of pain to the spinal cord in RSD (mitigating against surgery): wide dynamic range (WDR)
1948	Sunderland	Perpetuation of pain and RSD at spinal cord level: "turbulence phenomenon"
1955	Mitchell	Sympathetic preganglionic cell bodies in all levels of spinal cord
1957	Tracey	Postsympathectomy pain (also called sympathalgia pain to the spinal cord in RSD) mitigating against surgery
1964	Weirtz-Hoessels	Paresis and weakness of extremity due to RSD
1970	Akil	SIA (stress-induced analgesia) in rats achieved by endorphines
1971	Melzack	Biasing mechanism of pain in CNS perpetuating RSD pain
1971	Goldstein	Discovered opiate receptors in the brain

TABLE 1 (Continued)

Year	Author	Contribution
1973	Kleinert	"Variable pain syndrome" as sympatoms of RSD
1973	Duensing	Thermography in nerve injuries
1973	Bonica	Comprehensive 3-stage classification of RSD; early diagnosis critical in outcome of treatment
1973	Patman	Mimocausalgia
1974	Hannington-Kiff	Guanethidine regional block with up to 80% relief
1975	Lichtenstein	Loss of vascular tone, vasodilation, and bone resorption
1976	Wallin	Hyperpathic (sympathetic) pain is different from somatic pain; injection of sympathetic amines induces hyperpathic pain in causalgic limb but not in normal limb
1976	Kozin	Bilaterality in RSD; bone scan
1976	Travell	Defined trigger points and trigger point injections in management of RSD
1979	Moskowitz	Role of trigeminovascular structure in vascular headaches
1981	Kozin	Diagnostic value of scintigraphy, abnormal in 60% of RSD patient
1983	Poplawski	"The most important factor in predicting improvement was... less than 6 months between onset of RSD and the administration of therapy"
1984	Basbaum	Descending analgesic endorphin system from periaqueductal gray to spinal cord
1986	Ochoa	ABC phenomenon (angry backfiring c fibers as a source of pain and RSD
1986	Uricchio	Thermography in radiculopathy
1988	Roberts	Role of peripheral nervous system and CNS in pathophysiology of causalgia
1988	Wexler	Standardized thermography and its use in RSD
1988	Hobins	"Reflex sympathetic dysfunction"
1989	Yokota	Motor paresis and movement disorder due to efferent manifestation of RSD
1990	Schwartzman	Movement disorders due to RSD
1991	Stein	Peripheral release of lymphocyte-mediated endorphin originates an analgesic system that is in effect in all levels of CNS and PNS

TABLE 2
RSD Synonyms

Synonym	Author
Erythromelalgia	Mitchell (1864)
Causalgia	Mitchell (1867)
Sudeck's atrophy	Sudek (1900)
Traumatic angiospasm	Morton and Scott (1931)
Traumatic vasospasm	Lehman (1934)
RSD	Evans (1947)
Mimocausalgia	Patman (1973)
Minor causalgia	Homans (1940)
Shoulder-hand syndrome	
Chronic traumatic edema	
Sympathalgia (usually referred	Tracey, 1957;
to postsympathectomy pain)	Raskin, 1974
Posttraumatic pain syndrome	
Hyperpathic pain	
SMP (sympathetic mediated pain)	Lofstrom et al. (1988)

TMJ disease is commonly a manifestation of RSD, and infrequently due to temporomandibular joint pathology. TMJ can cause RSD, and vice versa

Thoracic outlet syndrome (TOS) is rarely an entity in itself. More commonly what is called TOS is a manifestation of referred pain from cervical spine pathology. The same pathology causes pain as well as spasm in muscles of thoracic outlet triangle. The muscle spasm produces a classic TOS. TOS surgery obviously will not correct the cervical spine pathology

In rare cases the thoracic outlet spasm of muscles (especially scalenus anticus) is solely due to efferent manifestation of RSD (see Chapter 5)

may culminate in the disastrous procedure of amputation. Amputation not only does not cure RSD, but it can be the cause of RSD.[253]

In 1851 the French Father of Physiology, Claude Bernard,[427a,427b] described the role of the sympathetic nervous system in preservation of *milieu interne*. He was the first to describe the sympathetic nervous system as being responsible for temperature regulation and regulation of the internal balance in the body.

The first report of clear-cut pathologic sympathetic dystrophy was made by the american neurologist, S. Weir Mitchell,[228,230] who reported for the first time the victims of sympathetic dystrophy on the wounded soldiers of the Civil War. He colorfully called this condition erythromelalgia, implying reddish sick pain.[230] In 1867 he described the condition in more detail and called it causalgia.[228]

Sudeck, in 1900, reported the association of osteoporosis and bone destruction with vascular changes in the extremities due to sympathetic due to sympathetic dystrophy.[359]

In 1916 the French surgeon Leriche[189] performed the first sympathectomy. Since 1923 when Orbeli described the antifatigue effect of sympathetic nerves on muscles on the extremities (Orbeli effect), other authors have reported dystonias, muscle spasm, and paresis of the extremities due to RSD (Weirtz-Hoessels[414]). Orbeli[259] associated sympathetic dystrophy with autonomic nervous dysfunction for the first time in 1926.

Zur Verth (as quoted by Escobar[94]) in 1929 pointed to the nervous emotional connotations accompanied by the type of pain associated with sympathetic dystrophy, and he called the condition peripheral acute trophoneurosis.[94]

In 1932 Hisey[469] demonstrated the role of the brain in control of ovulation. This was the foundation for modern neuroendocrinology, proving the brain is a glandular structure controlling the endocrine system.

Lehman in 1934 emphasized the importance of vasospasm in this condition and called the condition traumatic vasospasm.[94]

DeTakats (1937) emphasized the reflex nature of the condition and called it reflex dystrophy of the extremities.[79]

Homans[146] in 1940 divided the causalgias into major and minor. He demonstrated that the major causalgias were secondary to nerve damage, whereas minor causalgias lacked peripheral nerve damage as the etiology of reflex sympathetic dystrophy.

Livingston[197] in 1943 described the key pathogenic phenomenon of vicious circle as the mechanism of development of reflex sympathetic dystrophy secondary to disuse and inactivity. This principle of vicious circle is the key to proper treatment of RSD with physiotherapy.

Steinbrocker in 1947, by coining the terminology **reflex neurovascular dystrophy**, pointed to the chief features of trophic changes, neurovascular influence of sympathetic nervous system, and the reflex mechanism of the disease.[354]

In 1947 Evans first used the most popular terminology, reflex sympathetic dystrophy syndrome (RSDS), which has become universal in describing the illness.[95]

However, this terminology does a disservice to the illness by implying that the disease is invariably advanced, resulting in dystrophic changes in the extremity. It was in the late 1980s when Dr. G. Hobins from Madison, Wisconsin, introduced the terminology **reflex sympathetic dysfunction**. This is a more accurate terminology since it refers to the fact that the disease can be diagnosed with the help of thermography before it causes dystrophic changes.

Nathan[242] in 1947, Sunderland and Kelly[362] in 1948, and Roberts[301] in 1986 emphasized the influence of the spinal cord at multiple levels in transmission as well as perpetuation of the sympathetic pain. The Nathan and Roberts phenomenon explains why surgical intervention for RSD at the spinal cord level (tractotomy or nerve stimulation) is *doomed to fail*. Unfortunately, even up to the present time many surgeons have not heeded this important warning.

In 1967 Serre et al. introduced the term **reflex algodystrophy**, which emphasizes the importance of pain as the symptom of this disease.[335]

Akil et al.[462] in 1970 showed the role of **endorphines** in the important phenomenon of **stress-induced analgesia** (see Stress and RSD).

Melzack in 1971 introduced the *central biasing mechanism* in the phenomenon of perpetuation of chronic pain and RSD.[221] This central biasing mechanism shows the modulation and feedback of chronic pain and RSD up and down the central nervous system from the spinal cord all the way to the high centers of the brain.

Again, this mechanism is quite an important lesson which should discourage any enthusiastic surgeon from trying to find an answer for relief of chronic pain or RSD by applying invasive procedures in the CNS. Chronic pain and RSD are too diffuse, too elusive, and one lesion or surgical disruption in one area of the peripheral or central nervous system cannot control such a diffuse phenomenon and is apt to fail.

In 1971 Dr. Avram Goldstein (Goldstein et al.[470]) filtered the blender-homogenized brain through a funnel-shaped filter. By passing different chemicals through this funnel filter, he noted that heroin would not pass through the filter 100% intact. The brain had receptors absorbing some of the heroin. This *lock and key phenomenon* opened the door to the presence of *endorphins* to the better understanding of pain and addiction.

Bonica in 1973[36] emphasized the differences among the three stages of reflex sympathetic dysfunction (Table 3).

The first stage is characterized by constant burning pain and surpasses the sympathetic dermatomes. It is aggravated by any form of emotional stress.

Bonica[36] emphasized that the *second stage* usually occurs between 3 and 7 months after the injury and is associated with less pain than stage one. The second stage is typically accompanied by vasoconstriction and coolness of the extremity. Bonica emphasized that the differ-

TABLE 3
Stages of RSD

Stage 1

R.S. Dysfunction	**Disuse**	**Ephaptic (Causalgia)**
Onset	1–3 months	2–8 weeks
Symptoms	Burning pain beyond the dermatomes (follows thermatomes)	
	Spasm and tendency for immobilization	

Stage 2

R.S. Dystrophy	**Disuse**	**Causalgia**
Onset	3–7 months	2–4 months
Symptoms	Vasoconstriction	
	Unilateral cold extremity	
	Hair loss	
	Tendency for weakness, tremor, and spasticity (flexed arm, extended leg)	

Stage 3

R.S. Atrophy	**Disuse**	**Causalgia**
Onset	Over 7 months	Over 4 months
Symptoms	Smooth glossy edematous skin	
	Pale or cyanotic skin	
	Lymphedema	
	Atrophy of distal muscles	
	Spasm, dystonia, tremor	

Stage 4[a]

	Disuse	**Causalgia**
Onset	Several months to years	A few months
Symptoms	Loss of job and spouse in rare advanced severe cases	
	Unnecessary surgery	
	Orthostatic hypotension	
	Hypertension	
	Heart attack	
	Neurodermatitis	
	Angiectasis	
	Depression, death due to suicide	

[a]   This is an additional classification.

ence of temperature between the two limbs is not as obvious in stage three as it is in stage two.[36] This fact is quite essential, pointing to the bilateral nature of RSD in advanced stages.

In the *third stage*, the condition is so advanced that it is easily diagnosed with smooth and glossy skin, pale or cyanotic and dry skin, brittle nails, hypertrichosis, osteoporosis, and pathologic fractures. Any lay person can diagnose this stage, but it is too late for treatment.

Eventually, the untreated or passively treated patients in the third stage of RSD end up with depression, suicide, or unnecessary surgery with further aggravation of pain.

This disastrous stage — which we call *stage four* — can be properly prevented and aggressively treated.

In the same year (1976) Travell[377] made a major contribution to management of RSD by showing the importance of trigger points in the perpetuation of chronic pain. Travell also pointed to a practical and effective mode of therapy for trigger points. This is in the form of trigger point injections, which can be done with anesthetics, antiinflammatory medications, or just needle stimulation at the site of the trigger point.

The trigger point is a reflection of referred pain, which is typical of chronic RSD. The trigger point had been recognized long before Travell emphasized the significance of it in management of RSD. As early as the 1940s, experienced orthopedists in Europe, Canada, and the United States applied trigger point injections for management of bursitis and other forms of referred pain. However, Travell's contribution was threefold: she showed the significance of

(1)   certain common trigger point regions,
(2)   trigger points in the management of RSD, and
(3)   trigger point injections in physiotherapy for RSD.

The trigger point injection is not just a temporary relief of pain or placebo effect. It disrupts and interferes with the repetitive input of hyperpathic pain to the spinal cord with secondary wide dynamic range stimulation of the spinal cord. In this regard, it is very similar to acupuncture, and practically on the same basis can break down the vicious circle of conditioned reflex of chronic pain.

The trigger point also results in inhibition of efferent motor dysfunction of RSD with resultant relaxation of the muscles in the distal portion of the involved extremity.

Bernstein et al., in 1978, reported the propensity of children for development of RSD and emphasized the better prognosis among children than in adults regarding the outcome of RSD.[27]

It is true that not only children but uneducated patients as well as patients from primitive cultures rich in superstition tolerate chronic pain and especially RSD very poorly. For example, Haitians tolerate RSD more poorly than other cultures. Some of it is the difficulty to make a child or a superstitious person understand that the treatment requires infliction of pain by exercise or sympathetic nerve block, and some of it is because RSD is so difficult to understand that even the majority of physicians do not understand the pathologic mechanisms of RSD, let alone children and uneducated individuals.

The above does not implicate any racial tendency or, for that matter, any preexisting psychopathology in pain development.

Children may tolerate RSD poorly, but they recover from it quickly. The surge of growth hormone and other hormones during adolescence has a strong healing effect on neurologic injuries.

Kozin et al., in 1977, pointed to the usefulness of scintigraphic tests in early diagnosis of RSD. Scintigraphic radioisotope bone scanning can be helpful in the diagnosis of RSD.[177]

In 1981 Kozin emphasized the fact that bone scanning quite frequently shows abnormality bilaterally,[178] reflecting the bilateral nature of sympathetic innervation, which has been emphasized by Bonica.[36,37]

Radioisotope bone scan test is second only to thermography in its sensitivity in the diagnosis of RSD. However, as RSD becomes chronic, the bilateral representation of RSD becomes more obvious. This bilaterality is not only in the form of pain and edema, but also in the form of abnormal radioisotope uptake in both extremities rather than one extremity.

In the early stages of RSD due to vasoconstriction, the bone scan may show false lateralization and show the abnormality in the opposite extremity. Later in subacute stages, the abnormality is seen bilaterally. In stage three or chronic stages of RSD, the bone scan becomes more obvious and more abnormal on the side of the traumatized extremity. As a result, serial bone scanning on the same patient can be quite confusing and can show different pictures at different stages of RSD.

Lankford and Thompson[186] in 1977 considered the physiological premorbid state of the patient as the cause of RSD. However, later reports[378] considered the pathological changes in

RSD as an effect and byproduct of the painful neurovascular changes in RSD rather than the cause of this condition.

In 1986 Ochoa[249] discovered the ABC (angry backfiring c fibers) phenomenon. This phenomenon is the key pathologic factor in the development of RSD in scarred areas of peripheral nerves damage. This form of RSD, also called ephaptic RSD, is less common than the disuse RSD, but because of the angry backfiring c fibers, it is likely to persist and be quite intractable to treatment.

Finally, the history of accumulation of knowledge regarding RSD has had a close association and affinity with the major wars in the nineteenth and twentieth centuries. After the Civil War, World Wars I and II, Korean, Vietnamese, and Lebanese Wars, both surgical and medical studies were done on the subject of RSD. During and after World War II and following major wars, sympathectomy was hailed as a most effective treatment for RSD.

The succeeding civilian decades proved sympathectomy to be nothing but a temporary band-aid and a temporary palliation with excellent short-term results. Long term, sympathectomy proved to be a failure in the majority of RSD patients (see Chapter 13, Sympathectomy).

The contrast in treatment results between RSD during war and RSD during life is not only noted in the study of surgical treatment of RSD, but also in the medical treatment of RSD, and shows the same confusing and contrasting results. During the war in Lebanon, treatment with oral dibenzyline resulted in excellent relief of pain. Yet in civilian RSD patients, dibenzyline is not well tolerated, and the treatment is not as dramatically successful.

This contrast in war vs. civilian forms of RSD may be due to the fact that any treatment, be it surgical or medical, that takes the soldier away from the war zone may have a very strong psychological beneficial effect, hence, resulting in a happy ending. In addition, the war wounds are more likely to be acute with strong stress-induced analgesia (SIA) (see Chapter 4) overtone in contrast to complex chronic pain (CCP) of civilian injuries with strong stress-induced pain (SIP) overtone.

TRUTH IS THE ONLY SURVIVOR

RSD and its management are in an infantile stage. There is a lot to be learned regarding the mechanism and management of this very painful and unpleasant condition. It is one form of chronic pain that crosses the boundaries of "organic" vs. "functional" artificial lines. It is a subject that is hard to understand because it is at best a pathologic laboratory for application of neurophysiologic complex principles.

Because the subject of RSD is difficult to understand, it always carries with it a fiery emotional debate and disagreement. Debate and disagreement at the present time are reflected on the subject of the use of thermography in the diagnosis of RSD.

Infrared **thermography** (Figures 2 and 3) is the most sensitive test in the diagnosis of RSD. At present it should be almost exclusively used for diagnosis of RSD. It is not as accurate for other causes of pain such as radiculopathy of disc herniation. It addresses itself purely to temperature differences and subtle temperature gradients in different parts of the skin. In this regard, it gives quite a sensitive and accurate detail of the temperature pattern over the body and makes a good contrasting comparison in temperature changes on one side of the body versus the opposite side.

Thermography has become a hot subject of debate because it has been advocated as being useful in different kinds of illnesses. Obviously thermography is not useful in the diagnosis of motor nerve root dysfunction or even subtle sensory nerve root dysfunctions. It does not show disturbance of **dermatomal** patterns of sensory nerve dysfunction, but it does show **thermatomal** patterns of **sympathetic nerve** distribution. It shows the temperature changes in the distribution of sympathetic nerves that follow **vascular** structures to the extremities, and, as a result, it overlaps the dermatomal distribution of sensory nerves (Figure 4a). In this regard, it becomes confusing if it is applied to the side in which a nerve root is affected by any disease.

On the other hand, the tests that identify motor nerve root dysfunction (EMG/nerve conduction times) or sensory nerve dysfunction (somatosensory evoked potentials SSEP) are more sensitive than thermography in identifying nerve root abnormalities.

It is childish to try to compare thermography with tests that assess abnormalities that thermography cannot identify. It cannot be compared with MRI, EMG, or SSEP. On the other hand, it is obvious that the latter tests cannot identify **subtle temperature gradients** essential in the early diagnosis of RSD.

Thermography has one main use in diagnosis and management of chronic pain, and that is the **identification of RSD**. In this regard, no other test can match thermography.

There is little debate regarding nonspecific and false positive results of anatomical tests such as MRI (Table 16) and CT scan. However, whenever a neurophysiologic tool such as thermography or evoked potential test is applied in diagnostic medicine, it results in extensive debate, not because neurophysiologic tests are useless, but because they are hard to understand and not as easily depicted as a simple anatomical test.

It is quite similar to the debate between the missionary and the witch doctor in front of a tribe when the witch doctor proved that he knew more about science than the missionary by drawing a fierce-looking snake as opposed to the nice handwriting of the word "snake" by the missionary.

One fact is indisputable: every century the physicians look at their predecessors and consider them backward and barbaric only to fall prey to the successors of the next century who pass the same judgment.

Long-term study of medical history proves that truth is the only survivor.

2

The Role of Sympathetic Nervous System in Temperature Regulation

There is a stark contrast between anatomy and physiology of the sympathetic system.

The anatomy of the sympathetic system is quite primitive. The system is intermingled with almost amoebic-shaped paraspinal **ganglia** and **plexi** (Figure 34). This results in an inter-mingled anatomical system that sympathetically causes a diffuse complex sympathetic response. In rare cases, for example, **lumbar** sympathetic block results in the development of RSD in ipsilateral heretofore asymptomatic **upper extremity**. More frequently, sympathetic block gets rid of tremor due to RSD in one extremity, only for the **tremor** to appear in the heretofore asymptomatic **opposite extremity**.

In contrast, the sympathetic system has a most efficient physiologic function. If there is one function that exemplifies the role of the sympathetic nervous system (SNS), it is the function of preservation of **proper distribution of energy**, especially **heat**, in different parts of the body.

Its function is **economy in heat loss** and **preservation of energy**.

When an extremity becomes inactive, the sympathetic nervous system reflexly reduces **blood circulation** to the skin of the extremity. The resultant vasoconstriction in turn prevents unnecessary radiation of heat through the skin of the extremity. This is the key to understand-ing the complex and highly efficient function of the sympathetic nervous system.

As chronic and hyperpathic pain results in inactivity of the extremity, the **SNS reduces** the **skin circulation** at the expense of **increasing the deep circulation** of the extremity. This results in osteoporosis secondary to rapid washout of the blood through the bone marrow.

The vasoconstriction aggravates the hyperpathic pain, and the hyperpathic pain induces **inactivity**. The condition becomes worse with improper application of a cast, brace, or ice to the painful extremity. It is imperative for surgeons and emergency room physicians to recognize this paradoxical reflex of the sympathetic nervous system. If such a phenomenon is recognized, then deterioration of RSD can be arrested.

Whereas, in **somesthetic type of pain**, application of **ice** may be quite helpful, in nocicep-tive **hyperpathic chronic pain**, application of ice only aggravates and contributes to the development of RSD.

The same is true in hand surgery. **Unnecessary arthrodesis** of the wrist, **unnecessary exploration of the damaged sensory nerves** in the palm or dorsum of the hand, and unnecessary injections in the area of the **scarred nerve** tissue lead to disastrous results of aggravation of severe pain and RSD due to marked hyperactivity of sympathetic nervous system and aggravation of vasoconstriction in the extremity.

13

Claude Bernard,[427a,427b] the French Father of Modern Physiology, was the first (1851) to point to the role of the sympathetic nervous system in the regulation of the body's internal environment (*milieu interne*). Bernard's principle emphasizes the fact that the autonomic nervous system in concert with the somatic nervous system alerts the organism to noxious painful stimuli or temperature changes.

THERMAL CHANGES

Claude Bernard in 1878 demonstrated that temperature regulation is an integral part of maintenance of the *milieu interne* (internal environment) in warm-blooded animals. Bernard[427a,427b] demonstrated that the sympathetic nerves are essential for the above function.

Sewall and Sanford[448] and Pickering and Hess[449] showed **bilaterality of the function** of the SNS in temperature regulation and its **dependence on an intact central nervous system** for temperature regulation. The thermoregulatory function is bilateral as well as **simultaneous** in the **upper and lower extremities** (Gibbon et al.[450]).

The effectors of temperature regulation are in sympathetic distribution both peripherally in the skin (Pickering[452]) and centrally in the CNS (Cranston,[451] Appenzeller,[453] and Appenzeller[441]).

The measurement of body temperature in disease is not new and has been utilized as far back as the history of medicine can be detected.

Saidman in 1949[312] and Stary in 1956[353] reported the temperature changes in as small fractions as 0.5–0.7°C to be diagnostic of disease.

The central temperature regulation is achieved by the hypothalamus through the sympathetic nervous system both centrally and peripherally.[1,20,21,23,50,58,59,101,103,104,106,121,153,161,167, 168,171,180,181,217,220,237,256,281,297,316,352,356,380–382,408,410]

In the hypothalamus the heat-sensitive neurons stop firing when the preoptic nucleus detects an increase in heat in the cerebral blood flow. This secondarily causes inhibition of the sympathetic neurons in the posterior hypothalamic region. The inhibition leads to vasodilation of the subcutaneous venous circulation. Vasodilation that occurs in the skin results in evaporation of heat.

The reverse is true in the case of a drop in temperature in the cerebral blood flow.

The sympathetic nervous system functions symmetrically, and the increase and decrease of temperature in normal conditions is influenced by the (Figures 2–4) sympathetic nervous system bilaterally.[112,155,203,285,381]

TEMPERATURE CHANGES IN RSD

Hyperactivity of the sympathetic system results in dermal vasoconstriction and reduction of skin temperature in symmetrical fashion (Figures 4–6).

In pathologic sympathetic hyperactivity (reflex sympathetic dysfunction) the temperature changes may be asymmetrical.

The two forms of RSD cause two different types of temperature changes:

1. In **synaptic dysfunction** (RSD of disuse aggravated by inactivity) there is a concentric reduction of temperature that is more prominent on the pathologic side (injured extremity) (see Figure 13b).
2. In ephaptic RSD (due to scar of peripheral nerve) the pathologic sympathetic dysfunction is not simply exerted through the synaptic cleft. Instead, it is caused by peripheral nerve damage. The damage causes increased firing at the distal synapse, and transaxonal electrical stimulation to adjacent damaged nerve fibers.

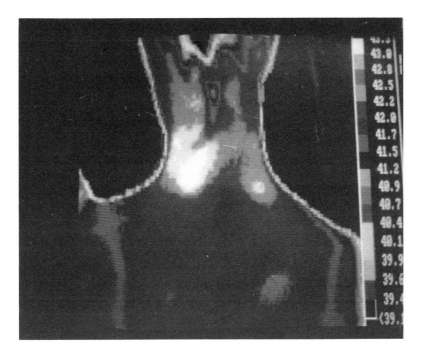

FIGURE 2a. Persistent left posterior cervical pain after C4–5 disc removal. RSD left upper extremity. Trigger point injections at left C4–5 interarticular region provided marked relief of pain. See also color plates following page 42.

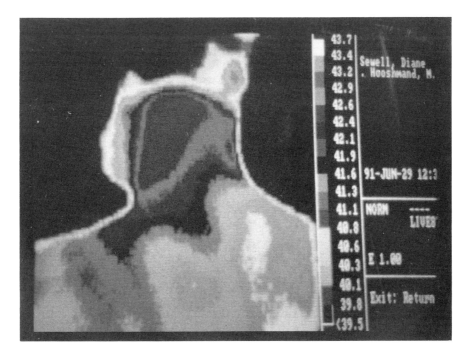

FIGURE 2b. Right cervical paraspinal trigger point (cold spot) at the C5-6 level. The corresponding normal side shows a reflex hyperthermic response. Three trigger point injections at the right C5–6 paraspinal region resulted in complete relief of pain. See also color plates following page 42.

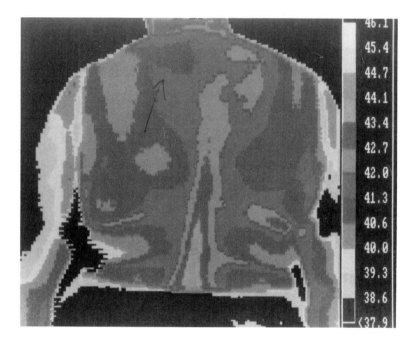

FIGURE 3. A cold spot over left trapezius muscle region in a patient suffering from left C4 and C5 nerve roots contusion, left shoulder-hand syndrome, and left upper extremity RSD. See also color plates following page 42.

This electric short — which bypasses normal synapse — is termed **ephapse*** which results in ephaptic transmission (Figure 14).

The **focal nerve damage** (ephapse) results in an island of turbulence and increased temperature in an already cold RSD extremity (Figure 5b1 and 5b2).

The **human skin**, the largest organ of the body, is an efficient thermoregulator. Efficacy of the body's thermoregulation by the skin is within the 95 percentile rate of perfection.

If the body does not emanate heat through the skin, the generation of the heat in the body can cause fever, central nervous system damage, and death. As the body is exposed to an increase in the external (ambient) temperature, the skin accelerates heat loss. As the body is exposed to cold temperature, the body tends to preserve internal heat by vasoconstriction of the external dermis.

This constant balance of vasodilation (heat loss) and vasoconstriction (heat preservation) is regulated closely by the autonomic nervous system. The sympathetic nervous system stimulation enhances skin vasoconstriction on the one hand and bone and muscle vasodilation on the other. Inhibition of this system has the opposite effect.

The sympathetic nervous system works quite symmetrically on the two sides of the body, and any significant thermal asymmetry (0.5–0.9°C) on the surface of the skin points to dysfunction of this system. Normally the sympathetic nervous system quite consistently preserves this symmetry of temperature.[380]

Bedside evaluation of temperature differences between the two sides of the body using the clinician's tactile acumen detects temperature differences only in the 5–6°C range. This is in contrast to 1–2°C difference that is present in most sympathetic nervous system dysfunctions.

Thermography can detect the most subtle temperature changes between the two sides. Thermography, as a tool in the diagnosis of RSD, is considered far superior to other tests (over 90% accuracy) compared to bone scans (over 50% accuracy) in the assessment of temperature

---

* Ephapse refers to a pathologic electric short in nerve fibers. This is in contrast to synapse, which avoids any electric short by buffer zone of synaptic cleft.

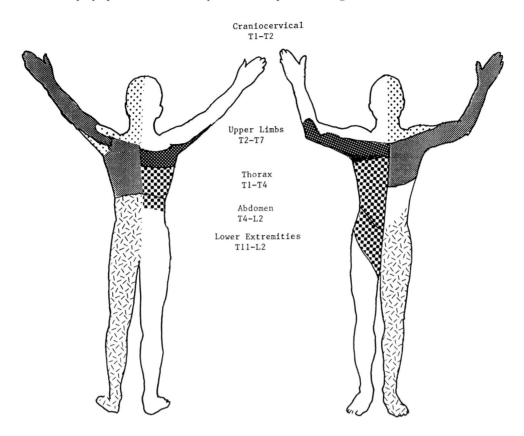

Craniocervical
T1–T2

Upper Limbs
T2–T7

Thorax
T1–T4

Abdomen
T4–L2

Lower Extremities
T11–L2

FIGURE 4a. Damage to the peripheral sympathetic nervous system (SNS) does not follow peripheral nerve dermatomes. It follows thermatomes: autonomic nerves that surround and follow the arteries and end up in sympathetic ganglia. They enter the spinal cord as follows: for head and neck, at T1–T2 levels of spinal cord; for upper extremities, at T2–T7 levels; for thorax, at T1–T4 levels; for abdomen, at T4–L2 levels; for lower extremities, at T11–L2 levels.

changes accompanying chronic pain.[409] Its use is practically limited to autonomic system evaluation.

The autonomic temperature changes that occur pathologically are usually either hot or cold areas (Figures 2 and 3). Both increases and decreases of subcutaneous temperature have been reported in RSD (Figures 5 and 6).

SYNAPTIC (DISUSE) RSD

The RSD of disuse, which is the most common type of RSD, results in temperature changes (usually reduction of temperature) in a thermatomal fashion. Thermatome is not exactly the same as sensory dermatome, but it more closely follows the autonomic sympathetic nerve distribution of the skin and blood vessels (Figures 4a, e, and f). The temperature changes are in a concentric symmetrical fashion with decreasing radiation from the proximal to the distal part of the extremity. This is in contrast with abrupt temperature changes seen in scleroderma (Figure 26).

In the first few days after an acute injury due to a trauma/shock to the SNS, increased skin temperature may develop. Within a few days, the skin temperature may drop below normal. This is subsequently followed by a decrease in temperature.

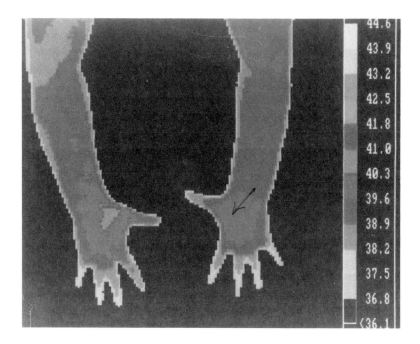

FIGURE 4b. Left C8 nerve root contusion after cervical sprain. EMG: moderate neurogenic changes in left C8 nerve root distribution. MRI is normal. Thermography shows reduction of temperature in left radial sensory nerve distribution with reflex hyperthermia in the homologous area in the right hand. The thermatomal distribution transgresses the dermatomal limits of the left C8 nerve root. See also color plates following page 42.

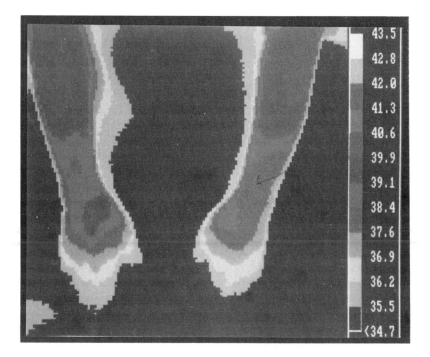

FIGURE 4c. RSD due to injury to the left hand. Note: (1) bilateral, symmetrical, concentric hypothermias, both hands; (2) thermatomal hypothermia, dorsum of left hand and forearm. The thermatomes do not follow the dermatomal distribution of peripheral sensory nerve roots.

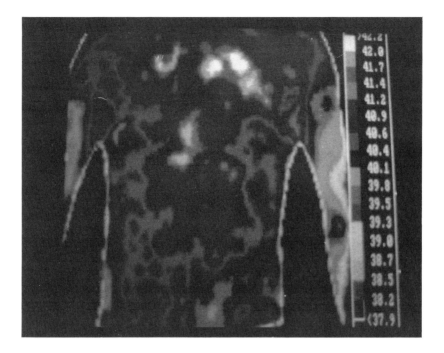

FIGURES 4d AND e. Electrical injury to left hand causing damage to C6, C7, and C8 sensory nerves and severe RSD over the left upper extremity. The hyperthermia over the anterior chest wall — more on the left side — is a common finding in such patients. This corresponds with thermatomal distribution of sympathetic nerves at the point of entrance to the thoracic spinal cord. Chest wall pain is also a common complaint in such patients. Neurologic examination invariably shows a band of mild sensory loss at T3-T4 levels on the chest wall. Somatosensory evoked potentials point to spinal cord dysfunction in these electrical injury patients. See also color plates following page 42.

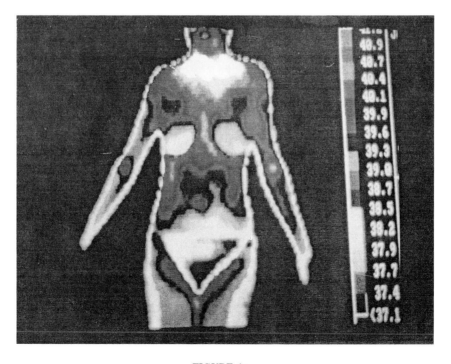

FIGURE 4e

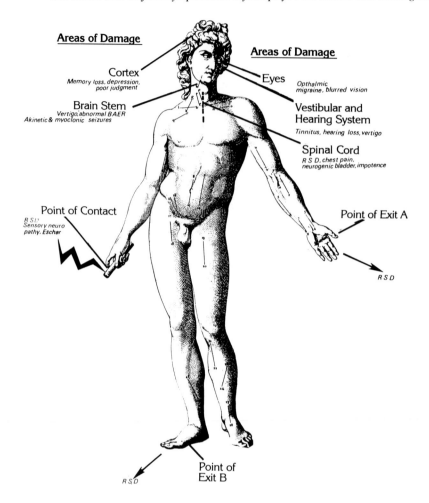

Areas of Damage

Cortex
Memory loss, depression, poor judgment

Brain Stem
*Vertigo, abnormal BAER
Akinetic & myoclonic seizures*

Areas of Damage

Eyes
*Opthalmic
migraine, blurred vision*

Vestibular and
Hearing System
Tinnitus, hearing loss, vertigo

Spinal Cord
*R S D, chest pain,
neurogenic bladder, impotence*

Point of Contact
*R S D
Sensory neuro
pathy. Eschar*

Point of Exit A

R S D

Point of
Exit B

R S D

FIGURE 4f. Damage to sympathetic nerves due to electrical injuries follows the wall of arteries and enters the spinal cord through the sympathetic ganglia. The damage ascends to the brain stem (vertigo) and limbic system (depression and memory loss). Areas of maximus injury: thoracic spinal cord, limibic system, and pain pathways. Note hyperthermia and sensory loss in the distribution of the upper thoracic nerve roots seen in Figures 4d and 4e (also see electrical injuries).

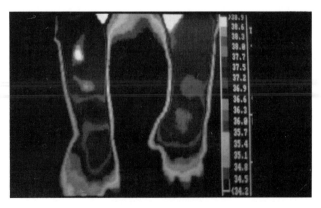

FIGURE 5a. Industrial injury causing right forearm causalgia. Note: (1) focal hypothermia in two areas of the causalgia, dorsum of right forearm. (2) Distal hypothermia over radial nerves distribution, left hand. (3) Symmetrical hypothermia, fingers of both hands. See also color plates following page 42.

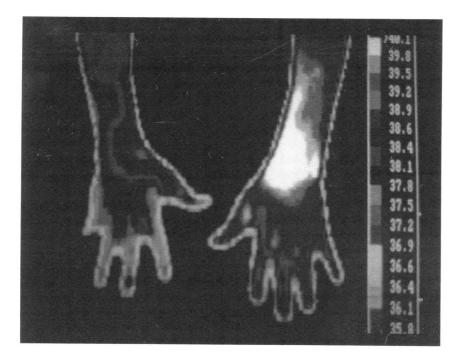

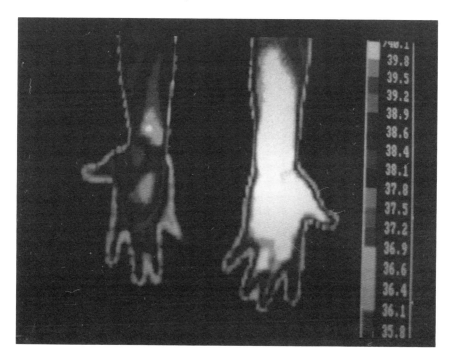

FIGURE 5b. Industrial crush injury to palmar and dorsal aspects of the right hand and right forearm. Ephaptic (causalgia) injuries show focal hyperthermia. The rest of the involved extremity is cold. Three weeks after the accident, the opposite extremity shows a compensatory reflex hyperthermia. See also color plates following page 42.

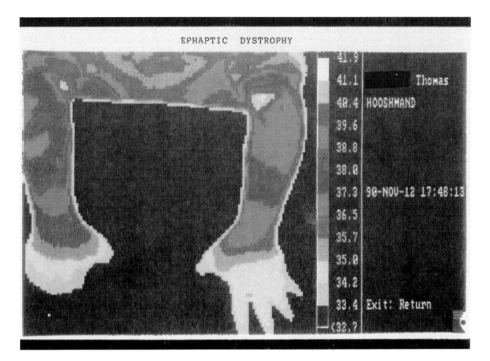

FIGURES 5c AND d. Industrial crushed sensory radial nerve injury, dorsum of right hand: (1) The causalgic (ephaptic) nerve injury shows hypothermia, dorsum of right hand; (2) the reflex contralateral disuse sympathetic dystrophy is concentric, symmetrical, and shows no focal thermatomal damage. See also color plates following page 42.

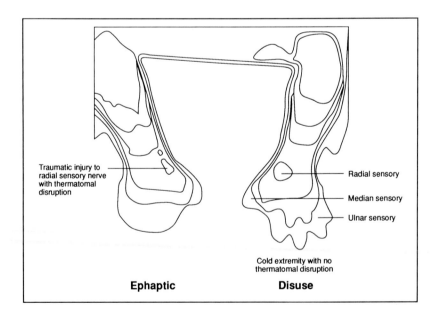

FIGURE 5d

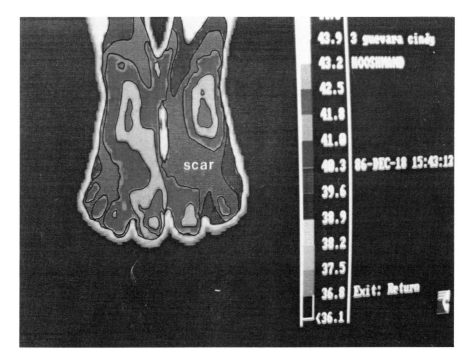

FIGURES 6a AND b. The most common form of civil causalgic (ephaptic) RSD occurs after injury to the dorsum of the left foot. This watershed area is tightly innervated by three different sensory nerves as demonstrated on b on the right foot sural nerve and superficial and deep peroneal nerves. A scar crossing these three watershed zones causes an electric short (ephapse in contrast to synapse) with resulant electrical firing and electrical discharge to the adjacent nerves. This scarred area of ephapse causes perpetuation of chronic pain and thermal changes as seen on the dorsum of the left foot in a. See also color plates following page 42.

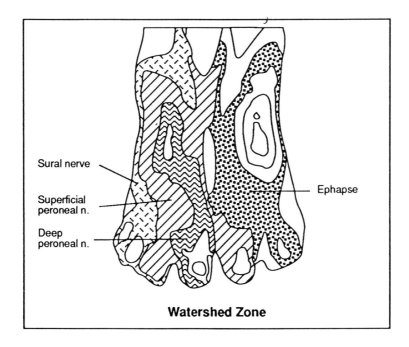

FIGURE 6b

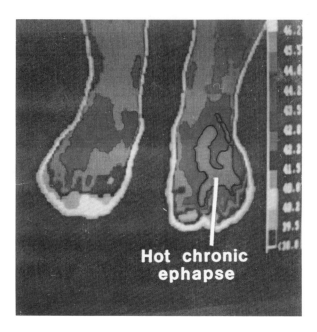

FIGURE 7. Twelve years after original injury and 7 years after lumbar sympathectomy, the area of scar (ephapse) shows Cannon phenomenon with focal hyperthermia and autonomous persistent pain. This patient required electroshock therapy to abort repeated attempts of suicide. The persistence of vasodilation may be partially the result of the release of nitrous oxide (NO) from the wall of damaged vessels. See also color plates following page 42.

TABLE 4
RSD Temperature Changes

Stage	Disuse	Ephaptic
1: First few days (see Table 3)	Both extremities warm	Both extremities warm
1: First few weeks	Both extremities cold	Scar cold, opposite extremity sympathetically warm (Figures 4c and 22)
2	Involved extremity cold	Scar cold, opposite extremity normothermic (Figure 5)
3: Early	As above	As above
4: Late and post-sympathectomy	Involved extremity warmer	Scar persists and is warmer than surrounding areas: Cannon phenomenon (Figures 4e–f and 7)

EPHAPTIC (CAUSALGIC) RSD

In the less frequent forms of RSD, ephaptic RSD and causalgia, months after the extremity becomes hypothermic, the scarred area of the damaged nerve becomes hyperthermic in relation to the surrounding cold skin (Figures 5–7; Table 4).

The temperature increase over the ephaptic scar is multifactorial in this situation, and is the result of damage to the sympathetic nerve fibers with resultant paralysis of sympathetic nerve fibers' function of heat preservation.

CAUSES OF HOT SPOTS

1. Damage to the sympathetic nervous fibers. Injury to the sympathetic nerve fibers results in paralysis of heat preservation in the area of the scar, as well as after sympathectomy. Years after sympathectomy, the scar area continues to be hyperthermic in relation to the surrounding intact skin. This is the result of the peripheral autonomous Cannon phenomenon (Figure 7) due to focal generation of norepinephrin and substance P. This is one of the reasons why sympathectomy fails in the long run.

2. Secretion of substance P, lactic acid, histamines, rogue oxygen, and disturbance of calcium efflux at cell membrane.

3. Ephaptic pathologic external reflexes in major or minor causalgias result in an electric short at the area of the scar with resultant increase in electrical discharge. This in turn results in mechanical increase of heat as well as secretion of painful substances (Figures 4c–f).

    This ephaptic electric short results in the phenomenon of deafferentation (Figure 8), which in turn causes perpetuation of pain with resultant spasticity, hypertonicity, tremor, and dystonia. The increased muscle activity contributes to the localized heat accompanying the ephaptic RSD injury.

4. In addition, the above-mentioned **deafferentation**. Lack of proper proprioceptive inhibitory input to spinal cord results in lack of inhibition of the anterolateral (intermediolateral) horn cells of the spinal cord due to the absence of proprioceptive input on these cells. This in turn results in vasoconstriction of the normal blood vessels surrounding the damaged area. This vasoconstriction causes an increase in heat differential between the abnormal skin, which is hot, and the surrounding normal skin that undergoes vasoconstriction, and as a result becomes quite cold.

5. Damage to the sympathetic nerve fibers at the area of damaged axons results in lack of norepinephrine secretion causing vasodilation and exacerbation and perpetuation of the injury (Figures 5a, b1, b2).

6. The extensive sympathetic activity in the surrounding normal skin not only causes vasoconstriction secondary to increased adrenergic activity but also results in postganglionic cholinergic activity in sympathetic nerves. This causes extensive sweating and evaporation of the heat in the area surrounding the nerve damage (Figures 4–6). This reflex heat loss in the area of nerve damage causes a relative increase of temperature with secondary pain generation and further deafferentation due to the fact that normal proprioceptive input does not inhibit the sympathetic nerve activity in the area of scar. This in turn causes more pain and a vicious circle.

7. **Nonsympathetic hot spots**. Finally, it should be noted that not every dermal hot spot on the skin is an ephaptic dystrophy phenomenon. There are many other causes of hot spots such as bed sores (where the skin becomes burned and destroyed due to inability of the skin to emanate heat), infections, gout, and immune inflammatory diseases (arthritis, lupus, polymyositis), neurodermatitis, and chemical irritants such as deodorants and perfumes.

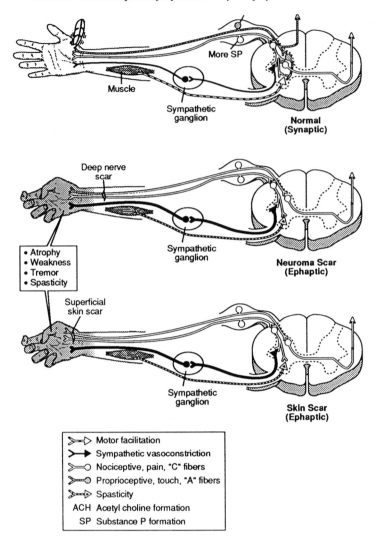

FIGURE 8. Diagram depicting deafferentation. Normally the proprioceptive impulses of touch and position senses inhibit the anterolateral horn cells of the spinal cord. This results in vasodilation and muscle relaxation. A nerve or skin scar changes the proprioceptive impulse to pain impulse. This deafferentation stimulates the anterolateral horn cells of the spinal cord with resultant vasoconstriction, cold extremity, and tremor or spasticity.

3
Anatomy of RSD

Whereas physiologically SNS is extremely efficient, anatomically it is quite vague and primitive in structure. The sympathetic nervous system is different anatomically from the somatic nervous system due to the fact that, in contrast with the sympathetic system, the somatic nervous system is quite clear-cut. In at least 95% of autopsies, it has a very consistent pattern.

On the other hand, the sympathetic nervous system (Figures 8 and 34) is not as clear-cut and consistent. Its anatomical structure is blurred by intermingling of nerve fibers in four large plexi, i.e., the **craniocervical, cardiac, celiac**, and **hypogastric**. In addition, there are several small intermediate and terminal ganglia present (Figure 34).

The sympathetic ganglia are positioned in the anterolateral area of the vertebral column. In the cervical spine region they are anterior to the transverse processes; in the thoracic spine region, they are anterior to the head of the ribs; in the abdominal region, they are lateral to the vertebral bodies; and in the pelvic region they are in front of the sacrum. The prevertebral ganglia up and down the spine have rich connection across the midline (Figure 34), and there is a tendency for fusion of the ganglia. As a result, there is no clear-cut single ganglion for every segment of the sympathetic nervous system.

There are three pairs of sympathetic ganglia in the cervical spine region, 12 in the thoracic spine and 4 in the lumbar spine, as well as 4 in the sacral spine region (Figure 34).

The preganglionic fibers mainly originate from the anterolateral horn cells of the thoracic spinal cord (Figures 9 and 10), but there is origination of other preganglionic fibers in the entire spinal cord. These points of origin are not as clear-cut as the preganglionic fibers leaving the thoracic and lumbar spinal cord. As these fibers leave the thoracic and lumbar spinal cord via the anterior nerve roots, they form white rami that connect to the chains of ganglia (Figures 9 and 10).

The **gray rami** that originate from these sympathetic ganglia carry the postganglionic nerve fibers back to the spinal nerve (Figure 8).

In addition, other preganglionic fibers travel up and down the sympathetic chain and connect the higher and lower ganglia (Figure 9).

This **diffused vertical connection** as well as across the midline connection of preganglionic nerve fibers results in a diffused, almost **amorphous sympathetic system**, which is not accurately amenable to surgical excision.

A spinal nerve originating from the spinal cord contains postganglionic sympathetic nerve fibers. These sympathetic nerve fibers are both **adrenergic (vasomotor)** and **cholinergic (sudomotor)**. The cholinergic fibers are responsible for the **autonomic control of the hair, sweating**, and **nails** growth (Figures 9 and 10).

As the **postganglionic fibers** travel down to the plexi, they follow different structures. The

27

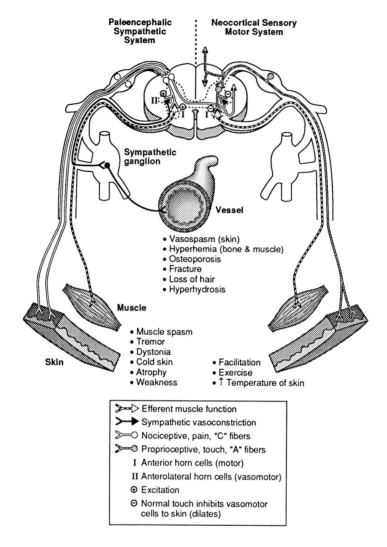

FIGURE 9. Proprioceptive input (right side of diagram) exerts inhibitory effect on anterolateral (intermediolateral) horn cells of the spinal cord with resultant inhibition of vasoconstriction and muscle spasm. Nociceptive stimulation of small C-fibers (left side of diagram) stimulates the anterolateral horn cells of spinal cord with resultant vasocontriction, muscle spasm, and cholinergic changes (hyperhydrosis and hair loss). See also color plates following page 42.

craniocervical postganglionic fibers traveling to the head and face follow the path of the arteries and are present mainly in the **periarterial connective tissue**.

The sympathetic nerves that follow the path of **visceral** (abdominal) and femoral plexi do not have an exact somatosensory pattern. Their **thermatomal distribution** is not exactly identical to the dermatomal distribution of the somatosensory nerves (Figure 4a).

The **abdominal viscera** receive the sympathetic fibers through the **coeliac plexus**. This plexus receives the preganglionic fibers in the **splenic nerves**, and the coeliac plexus supplies postganglionic sympathetic nerve fibers to the upper abdominal viscera (Figure 10).

What complicates the anatomical structure is that the sympathetic nervous system is also occupied by nerves from the parasympathetic nervous system. One example is the fact that the coeliac plexus recieves a major nerve branch from the **right vagus** nerve.

The most accessible anatomical structures for nerve block are the **stellate ganglion** in the base of the neck, the **coeliac plexus** anterior to the body of L1 vertebra, and the **lumbar sympathetic plexus**.

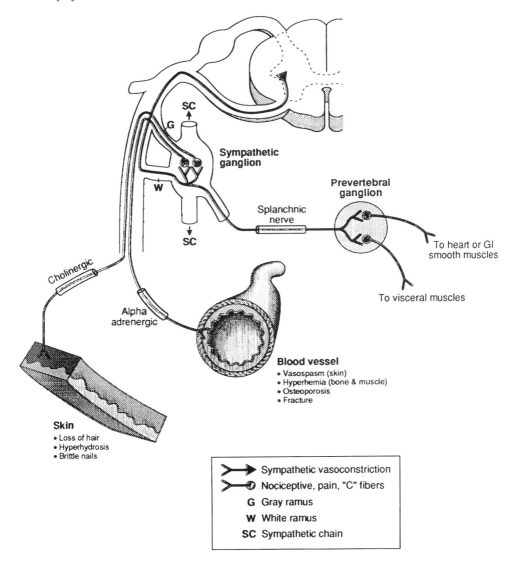

FIGURE 10. White and gray rami carrying pre- and postganglionic nerve fibers. Paravertebral ganglia carry visceral sympathetic nerve fibers. The coeliac prevertebral ganglion receives fibers from the vagus nerve as well.

The anatomy of sympathetic fibers — best detected by their thermal regulatory function — is not identical to the sensory system. The **thermatomal sympathetic system distribution** in many areas **transgresses the somatic dermatomes** (Figures 4a–e). This is especially so for the sympathetic nerve fibers from upper extremities which follow the arteries and end up in upper thoracic (T2–T5) levels of spinal cord (Figure 4a). Hence the frequent occurrence of chest pain in RSD of upper extremities.

CHEMICAL STRUCTURE OF THE SYMPATHETIC SYSTEM

The sympathetic system influences the control of temperature, vasoconstriction, and pain modulation from soft tissues in periphery up to highest centers of the CNS. This is a putative ascending/descending system that controls the above three essential functions.

Even lymphocytes in the areas of soft tissue injury influence pain by transmission of endorphins.[447]

The ascending system for relay of nociceptive pain is mainly influenced by concentration of substance P (sP), vasoactive polypeptide (VIP), and somatostatin in prevertebral ganglia and the sympathetic fibers (Hokfelt and Kellerth[482]).

The descending pain inhibitory system, originating from periaqueductal gray and ending in dorsal horn cell of spinal cord, mainly utilizes enkephalins for their inhibitory function. Somatostatin on the other hand seems to exert an excitatory efferent influence in the enteric portion of the sympathetic system (Elfvin[483] and Appenzeller[484]).

For more detail on the chemical anatomy of sympathetic system, see Chapter 4 (under "Chemicals Influencing Stress-Induced Analgesia (SIA)", and "Sympathetic Pain") as well as Chapter 7 (under "Vicious Circle").

CHEMICAL ANATOMY

The concept of sympathetic system functioning through dopamine-norepinephrine-generating nerves and parasympathetic system functioning through acetylcholingergic nerves, although true, is a marked oversimplification.

The same is true in regard to pre- and postganglionic α- and β-adrenergic sympathetic nerves: the pre- and postganglionic fibers may be located in PNS or CNS. The best example of the latter is brain stem dysfunction such as vascular headache or tremor responding to β-blockers (see Chapter 12, propranolol).

The SNS is modulated chemically through a maze of putative neuroendocrine systems such as substance P-enkephaline or sP-dynorphine and norepinephrine-endorphine putative systems (see Chapter 4, Table 5).

Besides the ubiquitous chemicals acetylcholine (AC) and norepinephrine, which are present at all levels of PNS and CNS of the sympathetic system, some of the other biogenic amines have a propensity for selective concentration in different areas of the SNS:

1. Serotonin is exclusively formed in brain, but through descending inhibitory pain fibers, the chemical is concentrated in substantia gelatinosa of trigeminal nerve and spinal cord.
2. Dynorphine is found in a higher concentration in PNS and in postganglionic visceral nerve endings of SNS.
3. Substance P (also see Chapter 7, substance P), another plentiful ubiquitous small polypeptide, is formed in all levels of CNS and PNS. However, it is mostly formed and accumulated in the posterior horn of gray matter of the spinal cord and migrated distally to peripheral somatic and sympathetic nerve fibers. Along with norepinephrine, it is a strong excitatory neurotransmitter for pain.

Substance P elevates prolactin. This elevation is clinically utilized to separate pseudoseizures from true major motor seizures (Hooshmand et al., Technical and Clinical Applications of TBM, 1989).

Substance P at the mesencephalic level is counteracted mainly by enkephalines. At the spinal cord and peripheral SNS level, the sp is counteracted mainly by dynorphin.

OTHER CLINICAL APPLICATIONS OF CHEMICAL ANATOMY OF SNS

Other than what is mentioned above, Chapter 7 (migraine and RSD) and Chapter 12 (management of RSD: ACTH, α- and β-blockers, and calcium channel blockers) summarize other applications of the chemical anatomy of SNS.

Surgically the diffuse bilateral representation of this system makes it a poor target for surgical application (see Chapter 12, sympathectomy).

In regard to tractotomy, anterolateral cordotomy, and rhizotomy, the records are even more disappointing. The procedures should be limited for only palliative application at late stages of cancer pain.

Nathan and Smith[491] studied the sympathetic changes after **anterolateral cordotomies**: clinical correlation of postmortem examination of the 88 patients studied revealed that the vasomotor and sudomotor sympathetic function was not abated and was only minimally diminished after hemicordotomy (hemisection of the spinal cord).

Their study revealed that the **sympathomotor fibers** are supplied from both sides of the spinal cord. The **vasomotor fibers** have a wider distribution than the sudomotor fibers. The **white matter** adjacent to the intermediolateral horn of the spinal cord contains the **efferent fibers** for **vasomotor control**, for **blood pressure control**, and for unconscious control of **defecation and micturition**. Section of this area has the side effects of **orthostatic hypotension**, **vasomotor paresis**, and **partial disturbance of thermoregulation**. In **cervical spinal cord**, section of the same area also results in **Horner's** syndrome. The same study[491] reported a young male who had undergone cordotomy, who had intact erection after manual or imaginary stimulation. Yet, the feeling of pleasure and the function of emission were lost. It is concluded that the **parasympathetic paths have remained intact**, but the afferent fibers for pleasurable sensation of emission are disrupted.

THREE-BUCKET-IMMERSION TEST

The studies of sympathetic anatomy and physiology reinforce the **bilateral distribution of sympathetic innervation**. A simple experiment that can be carried out with three buckets of water exemplifies the **symmetrical bilateral function of SNS**: immerse one hand in a bucket of cold water and the other hand in a bucket of warm water. After a few minutes the discomfort clears and the two hands adjust to their cold and hot environments. Then immerse the two hands in lukewarm water. The cold hand feels warm and the warm hand feels cold.

Then immerse both hands in a bucket full of ice and water. The hands feel very cold. After withdrawal, the **dominant (usually right) hand feels less cold than the left hand**. Thermography shows the left hand to be 0.5–1°C colder. Except for the dominant hand being more active and better adjusted to temperature change, the sympathetic system works symmetrically and very efficiently to adjusting to the temperature changes of the environment.

Anatomy and physiology of SNS are discussed in more detail in the following chapters.

4

Pathophysiology of the Sympathetic System

There are two types of pain: (1) *acute warning type of pain* that is brief, temporary, and benign. This pain is essential for survival, and is a warning of an acute and usually temporary assault to the system, e.g., acute appendicitis, attacks of angina pectoris, and acute pain after exercise; and (2) *complex chronic pain* (CCP), which is persistent and hard to control.

These two types of pain are transmitted and modulated through two different areas of the central nervous system and cause two different types of reflexes. Anatomically there are two opposing reflex systems that influence the temperature, sensation, and tonus of the extremities. The two opposing systems originate through different types of sensory nerve fibers.

The sensory nerve fibers in the proprioceptive system (somesthetic system) have a function that is quite in contrast with the nociceptive system.

LATERAL (SOMESTHETIC) SYSTEM

The sensory nerve fibers for proprioception (senses of acute somatic, larger fiber pain perception as well as touch and position) originate mainly from skeletal muscles, tendons, muscle spindles, and receptors in the skin. The majority of the proprioceptive sensory nerves (Figure 9) are relatively large (size A-α) with an average of 15 nm. The A-β cutaneous touch and pressure fibers average 8 μm in diameter, and the A-δ mechanoreceptors and pain receptors are 1–4 μm in diameter. The mechanoreceptors end up in the posterior horn and ascend in the dorsal column and pain receptors in the lateral spinothalamic tract (Figure 11).

The laterally positioned somatic (somesthetic) pain transmitted in A-δ and large c fibers is a high-threshold focalized somatotropic pain (Table 5). This is in contrast with the medially positioned nociceptive system, which is transmitted through small c fibers.

The somesthetic pain fibers carry discrete pain impulses. The impulses ascend through the lateral spinothalamic tract to the lateral nuclei of thalamus (VPL) and end up in the postcentral region of the rolandic fissure in the contralateral cerebral hemisphere (Figure 12).

The nociceptive (Figures 9–12) pain is a diffuse, alarming, unpleasant pain with a tendency for originating referred pain. It has a wide dynamic range (WDR) (Figure 11) of stimulation and activation in the spinal cord.[29,213] The nociceptive pain ascends through a multisynaptic system medially positioned in the brain stem and terminates in the medial nuclei of the thalamus. The impulses terminate bilaterally in the limbic system (frontotempororeticular regions).

The somesthetic fibers branch off at the dorsal horn of the spinal cord (Figures 9–11). These branches through the internuncial granular cells of the dorsal horn exert an inhibitory effect

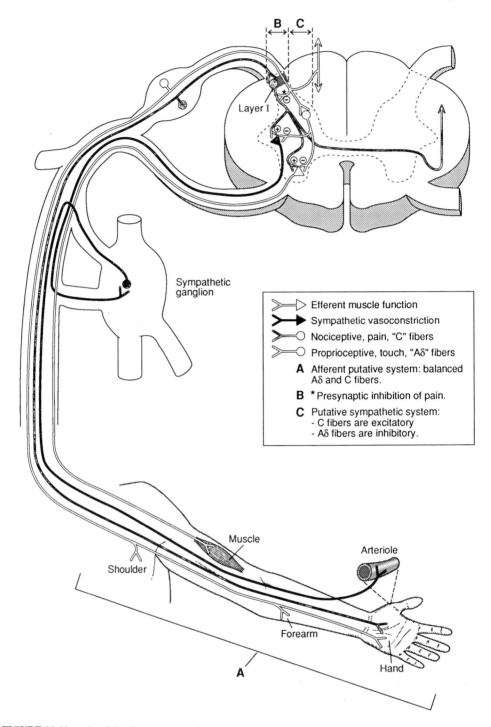

FIGURE 11. Normal peripheral nerves (A), substantia gelatinosa (B), and anterolateral horn cell level (C) putative systems. (A) A-δ and c fibers normally balance each other in peripheral nerves. (B) At layer 1 of the dorsal horn of the spinal cord the proprioceptive fibers inhibit the small c fibers input of pain. (C) At the anterolateral horn cells level the small c fibers exert excitatory and the A-δ fibers exert inhibitory influence.

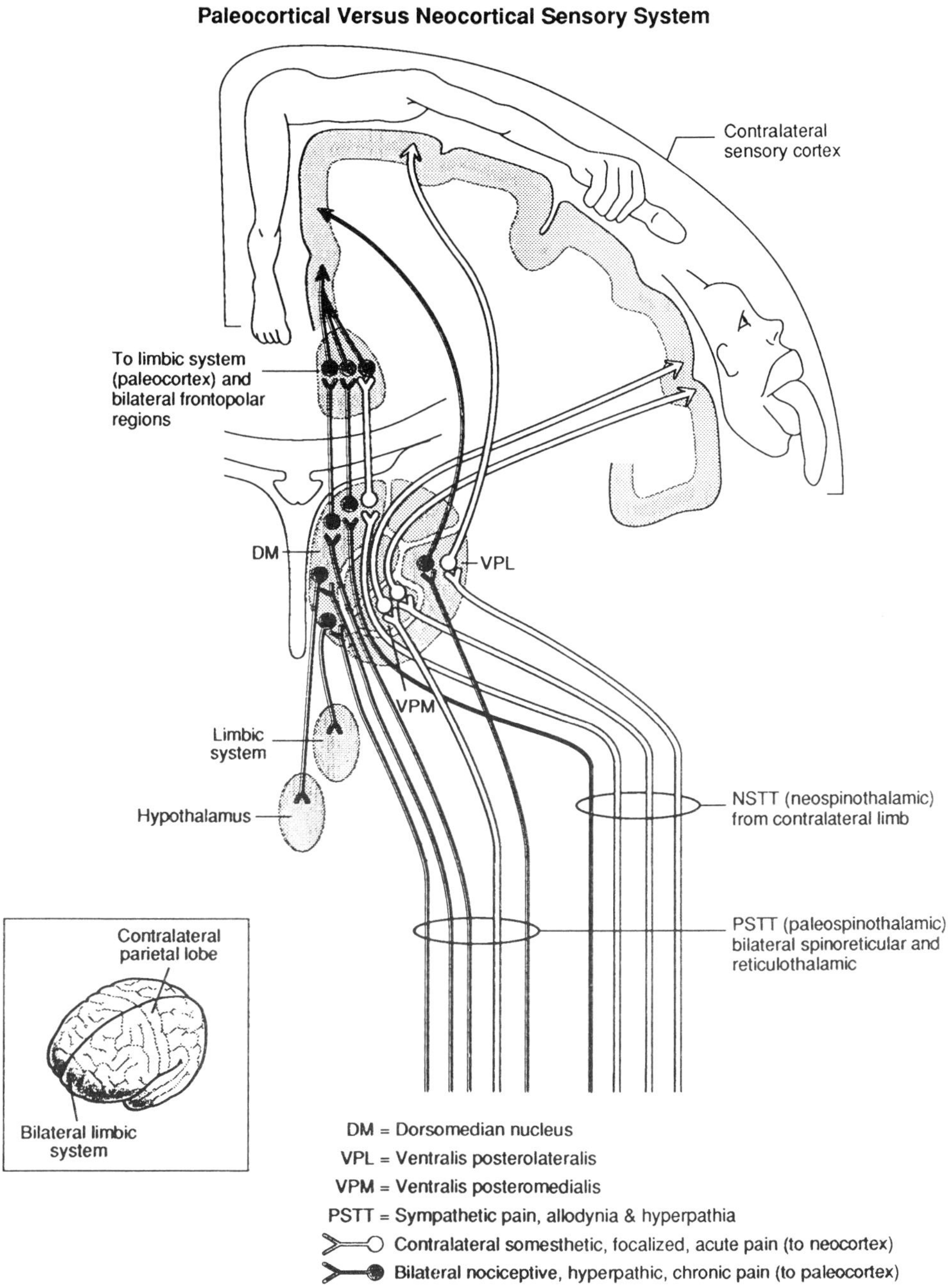

Paleocortical Versus Neocortical Sensory System

Contralateral
sensory cortex

To limbic system
(paleocortex) and
bilateral frontopolar
regions

DM

VPL

VPM

Limbic
system

Hypothalamus

NSTT (neospinothalamic)
from contralateral limb

PSTT (paleospinothalamic)
bilateral spinoreticular and
reticulothalamic

Contralateral
parietal lobe

Bilateral limbic
system

DM = Dorsomedian nucleus
VPL = Ventralis posterolateralis
VPM = Ventralis posteromedialis
PSTT = Sympathetic pain, allodynia & hyperpathia
Contralateral somesthetic, focalized, acute pain (to neocortex)
Bilateral nociceptive, hyperpathic, chronic pain (to paleocortex)

FIGURE 12a. Hyperpathic (red) pain system (paleocortical) is more multisynaptic (spinoreticulothalamocortical) and terminates in medial thalamic nuclei and bilateral limbic structures. The somesthetic (green) system (neocortical) contains less synaptic relays. It terminates in lateral nuclei of thalamus and in the contralateral somatosensroy parietal cortical region. See also color plates following page 42.

on vasoconstrictors and anterior horn nerve cells of proximal and distal portions of the spinal cord (Figures 9 and 11). The pain transferred in this system has its origin, in part, in the high-threshold pain fibers. The high-threshold cells are well suited for pain signal localization and accurate intensity identification.[308]

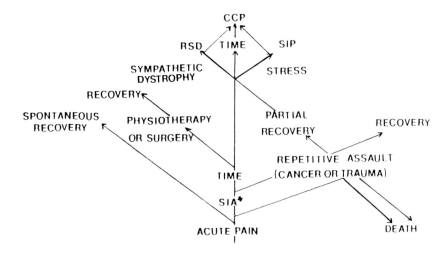

NATURAL DEVELOPMENTAL HISTORY OF PAIN

THREE DIMENSIONS OF COMPLEX CHRONIC PAIN

CCP: COMPLEX CHRONIC PAIN

RSD: REFLEX SYMPATHETIC DYSFUNCTION

SIP : STRESS INDUCED PAIN

SIA : STRESS INDUCED ANALGESIA

FIGURE 12b. Natural development of the history of pain. The majority of acute pain patients recover without any residual problems. Stress-induced analgesia (SIA) helps to enhance the complete recovery. RSD and SIP change the nature of chronic pain to complex chronic pain (CCP) which is more difficult to treat.

The somesthetic system is laterally positioned, hence the name lateral afferent system. The nociceptive pain terminates in the limbic system medially, hence the name medial nociceptive pain.

MEDIAL (NOCICEPTIVE) SYSTEM

Wallin et al.[397] demonstrated the pathologic nature of **nociceptive sympathetic pain** in contrast to **proprioceptive reflex pain**. In patients suffering from causalgia, hyperalgesia (hyperpathia) could be induced by locally injected sympathetic amines. Similarly treated subjects without a history of causalgia did not develop hyperpathia.[397]

The nociceptive nerve fibers responsible for perception of pain are of smaller size, and a majority of them are unmyelinated c fibers with a diameter of 0.5–1.5 µm.

These mainly unmyelinated c fibers originate from the skin, viscera, and wall of the blood vessels. These mechanoreceptors and nociceptors consist of the main nerve fibers of the sympathetic system, as well as sympathetic postganglionic nerve fibers.

As the pain fibers enter the dorsal horn of the spinal cord, they branch off to two main pathways (Figures 9, 11, and 12).

The first lateral path is the neospinothalamic tract (NSTT), mainly responsible for circumscribed feelings of touch and pain of a very localized nature. This tract ascends through the spinothalamic tract to the lateral nuclei of the thalamus, especially the VPL and VPM. From there, they synapse to the sensory nerve fibers that terminate in the somatosensory cortex (Figure 12).

The second path is the paleospinothalamic tract (PSTT) responsible for sympathetically mediated pain.

The pain, as it originates in the periphery and terminates in higher centers of the brain, is matched by endogenous analgesia: stress-induced analgesia (SIA) peripherally (mainly inhibited by dynorphin) as substance P is released due to the breakdown of tissues (Rubor, Rugeur, Duleor, and Chaleor). Lymphocytes originate endorphins (especially dynorphin)[477,478] to relieve the pain (Tables 5 and 5a). The endorphin release follows the path of pain centrally. A central descending endorphin originator analgesic system from periaqueductal gray to spinal cord counteracts the substance P-originated pain. Even this aspect of analgesia is different for hyperpathic vs. somesthetic pain (Table 5a).[476,477,479]

The PSTT is mainly responsible for stimulation of the sympathetic nervous system. The major contributors of this pathway are the wide dynamic range (WDR) nerve cells, which have a tendency for diffuse referred pain at the level of the spinal cord.[418] They ascend through the spinoreticular and spinomesencephalic tracts. From there, the pathway has synaptic relays to the medial thalamic nuclei (MT). From the MT, the fibers relay to the limbic forebrain (Figures 12a and 21) system and involve the entire limbic system in the brain stem, mesial frontal, and mesial temporal regions (Figures 12 and 21). This is a philogenetically older system and relays nociceptive painful impulses that are more nonspecific and more accompanied by allodynia (burning pain) and hyperpathia (intolerable pain).

In addition, the above-mentioned paleonociceptors (Figure 10) relay in the dorsal horn of the spinal cord and have an opposite effect on the anterolateral horn cells and anterior horn cells (Figure 10) of the spinal cord as compared to the proprioceptive system. They stimulate the anterior horn cells (Figures 10 and 11) to cause contraction of the muscles in the extremities, and this is in the form of a flexor withdrawal spasm from the source of pain (Figure 8). They also stimulate the anterolateral (intermediolateral) horn cells of the spinal cord with resultant vasoconstriction, sympathetic hyperfunction, and hyperpathia.

TABLE 5
Sympathetic Complex Chronic Pain (Sympathetic CCP)

	Hyperpathic or sympathetic pain (medial afferent system) (SMP)[b]	Somesthetic or somatic pain (lateral afferent system)
Phylogenetic	Mainly paleencephalic	Mainly neoencephalic
Cell type	Mainly wide dynamic range (WDR) cells (diffuse and referred pain	Mainly high-threshold cells (focalized, somatotropic pain)
Fibre size	Small C fibres with short relays in spinal cord to medial reticular, reticulothalamic, and thalamo-cortical tracts	Larger C and A-δ fibres in lateral spinothalamic and thalamocortical tracts
Spinal cord modulation	Layer 1 of dorsal horn — substance P vs. dynorphin putative system (sP, excitatory dynorphin inhibitory)	Layers 1–3 of dorsal horn NE sP vs. GABA and β-endorphin putative system (sP excitatory NE, and β-endorphin inhibitory
Thalamic site	Median and anterior nuclei	Lateral nuclei
Cortical	Bilateral prefrontal frontopolar, and limbic system	Contralateral sensory cortex and parietal lobe
Type of pain	Chronic pain	Acute pain
	Hyperpathic diffuse pain with perpetuation long after noxcious	Circumscribed focalized pain of shorter duration
Efferent	Flexion deformity, prolonged spasticity tremors, weakness of extremity, neurovascular dystrophy	Acute withdrawal followed by fatigue and poststimulus relaxation
Stress-induced analgesia (SIA)[a]	Not effective exhausted, with out of proportion response to pain	Effective helps suppress severe pain
Psychological	Depression, severe anxiety, inappropriate alarm	Acute temporary proportionate alarm
Thermography	Usually cold	Warm
Application of brace and cast	Aggravates	Helps
Application of ice	Aggravates	Helps
When indicated surgical exploration	Aggravates	Helps
Narcotics	See Table 5a	See Table 5a
Antidepressants	Help	Help in chronic stages

[a] Stress can raise the pain threshold through the descending inhibitory pathways in brain stem (both electrical and chemical, through secretion of dynorphin).[479,556]

[b] SMP = sympathetic mediated pain.

TABLE 5a
Opiate Receptors and Pain[476,477]

	Hyperpathic pain (sympathetic) (SMP)	Somesthetic pain
μ opiate receptors	No significant effect	μ opiate receptors activate G-protein G-protein in turn inhibits formation of cAMP Reduction of cAMP raises pain threshold
δ and κ opiate receptors	δ and κ opiate receptors relieve hyperpathic pain by blocking sympathetic postganglionic release of prostanoids and substance P	No significant effect
Lymphocyte-originated opioids	Peripheral release of opioids from lymphocytes; analgesia[477]	Analgesia

STRESS AND RSD

Stress is defined as any response influencing the internal harmony of the body, or as stated in the words of Claude Bernard, influencing the *milieu interne* or the balancing of the internal environment.

Although reliable for a general understanding of the various meanings of stress, its dictionary definition is wholly inadequate in providing a meaning of stress as the term is to be understood in the context of RSD.

In neurology, there are two terms, *stress* and *depression*, that are usually misunderstood. The term *depression* implies a reduction of the cerebral activity, whereas the opposite is the case in "depressed" patients. The depressed patient has a storm of cerebral activity that does not allow the victim to sleep properly. By calling the condition depression, one may imply that the patient is in need of a stimulant, which obviously is not the case. This misconception may wrongly result in the additional implication that antidepressants are "uppers", which again is a grave misrepresentation. *Stimulants* or *uppers* such as dextroamphetamine and Ritalin® have been tried on depressed patients with potential fatal complications of suicide and suicidal attempts.

Stress is another misunderstood term in medical practice. It often implies a pathologic connotation, as in the phrase, "any stress is bad". Nothing could be further from the truth. To place the term stress in a more proper and clinically usable context, we can describe two primary types of stress: *eustress* and *distress*. The stress that modulates the *milieu interne* may affect this balance of the internal environment in a beneficial manner or in a harmful fashion.

EUSTRESS

The stress that is beneficial was termed *eustress* by Dr. Hans Selye, a Canadian physician, in 1953. Some examples of eustress are

1. Pleasant physical exercise, such as recreation to balance the mental fatigue. Jogging, running, swimming, tennis, golf, etc., in moderation may reduce mental fatigue. Eustress helps normalize blood pressure, body weight, anxiety, and depression.
2. Pleasant mental exercise, such as good music, pleasant reading, biofeedback, meditation, prayer, good companionship, playing a relaxing game of cards, etc. The mental eustress balances the stress of excessive physical exercise and has similar beneficial effects on life as mentioned above.
3. Good sex, good food (see 4-F diet, Chapter 12), and proper natural sleep, that is sleep not induced by drugs.

DISTRESS

Distress is quite distinguishable from eustress in that it is a harmful disturbance, an imbalance of the internal system (*milieu interne*).

Any form of eustress carried out in excess or to the extreme changes into distress.

Other noteworthy examples of distress are

1. Bed rest to an excess. Excessive bedrest disturbs the immune system and creates a predisposition to disease. For example, excessive bedrest is very harmful to patients suffering from chronic pain, especially back pain as well as RSD.
    Late ambulation after surgery or after physical trauma causes obvious complications of emboli, delayed recovery, and superimposed illnesses.
2. Excessive exercise ("the Fixx phenomenon") is the best example of this distress. Jogging stimulates endorphins, and this results in a pleasant feeling (euphoria). Excessive jogging results in distress and may even result in heart attack.

3.   Improper food (see Chapter 12, section on Diet). The food consumed in the civilized world is more likely to be a distress than a eustress. A three-martini lunch followed by good wine and a steak full of fat and tyrosine certainly will not constitute eustress. The harms and distress of such a feast are self-explanatory.

4.   Iatrogenic medicine: that which does not readily lend itself to objective medical analysis imposes the greatest burden of care on the medical practitioner. It is no surprise that iatrogenicity is so commonplace in the field of pain in general, and RSD in particular since the subjective nature of the problem may lead so easily to misdiagnosis and, consequently, to mistreatment. The iatrogenic factor is nowhere more harmful in medicine than in the area of chronic pain. Other noteworthy examples of distress include prescribing bedrest for chronic pain, advocating inactivity and lack of exercise and physiography in RSD, and prescribing narcotics and BZ tranquilizers in chronic pain patients, especially those identified as suffering from RSD. Although these measures may appear warranted, they lead to disastrous results (see Chapter 12, Management of RSD).

Distress complicates chronic pain and results in complex chronic pain (CCP), which is difficult to treat.

PAIN AND STRESS

Pain is the common thread that weaves all the medical disciplines — medicine, dentistry, osteopathy, or chiropractic — together.

Pain is multidimensional (Figures 12a and 12b). In its most common form, acute pain, it is a simple somatic defense of transient nature. Acute pain is by and large harmless and benign. Cancer is the main exception, because it results in relentless destruction and longstanding repetitive acute pain.

Chronic pain has a tendency to persist long after the occurrence of the original noxious injury. Chronic pain in and of itself need not be miserable or intractable. Normal older people often wake up with some chronic aches and pains.

When chronic pain becomes complicated, it becomes hard to control. The complex chronic pain (CCP) adversely stimulates multiple areas of the nervous system. This multidimensional aspect of chronic pain taxes the patience of the clinician.

The temporal factor (chronicity) is not enough to qualify the pain as complex (CCP). Chronic pain complicated by one or more of the following factors passes for CCP:

1.   Involvement of the sympathetic system and the resultant abnormal vicious circle of vasoconstriction, inactivity, and perpetuation of pain due to reflex sympathetic dysfunction (RSD).

Chronic pain (CP) + RSD = CCP

2.   Depression in the form of emotional exhaustion and insomnia, usually due to longstanding use of narcotics or benzodiazepines and at times due to social and financial difficulties, can change the pain to CCP.

CP + Depression = CCP

3.   Stress-induced pain (SIP) due to distress of inactivity or other pathologic stressful factors is the opposite of stress (eustress)-induced analgesia (SIA).
      Eustress is discussed in detail in this book (Figures 12a and 12b).

$$CP + SIP = CCP$$

4. Aggravation of CP with central or peripheral nerve damage and scar is enough to cause CCP. A neuroma (e.g., phantom pain), a scar in the brain stem or thalamus, or a scar in a peripheral nerve (e.g., ephaptic causalgia or nerve contusion), changes CP to CCP.

$$CP + Neuroma\ or\ nerve\ contusion = CCP$$

The complex chronic pain (CCP) in contrast with the acute or chronic pain mainly stimulates the limbic system through the paleospinothalamic tract, discussed in detail in this book. This stimulation results in panic, depression, and low threshold for pain.

Reflex sympathetic dysfunction (RSD) is a form of CCP that mainly stimulates the limbic system and causes highly emotional hyperpathic pain (Figures 12a and 12b).

STRESS-INDUCED ANALGESIA (SIA)

Fortunately, the body is endowed with its own balancing system, albeit an imperfect one. This autogenerated response mechanism is known as stress-induced analgesia (SIA).[38] The shortcoming of this natural defense to pain is its inability to endure. As SIA is demanded for protracted periods, it eventually becomes exhausted with resultant aggravation of chronic pain. SIA is effective in suppressing pain temporarily.

Besides extensive experimental research confirming the efficacy of SIA,[38] there are clinical conditions that are best explained by SIA: a painful superficial laceration of a finger is relieved by exerting a strong pain, i.e., biting the finger. During war, soldiers are known to be totally unaware of large wounds or loss of a part of a limb while the battle is underway.

SIA (Figures 12a and 12b) is a descending putative system that exerts supraspinal modulation of pain at the dorsal horn level of the spinal cord.[38]

Distress stimulation of both pituitary and adrenal medullary originated β-endorphins and enkephalins causes excessive activation of dopamine and norepinephrine.

This putative system stimulates rostral ventromedial (RVM) nuclei of medulla, which in turn exert both inhibition (Basbaum[479]) of pain (enkephalin fibers) and excitation of pain (substance P and norepinephrine) on dorsal horn wide dynamic range (WDR) cells. SIA protects the individual against the harmful effects of excruciating pain.

This SIA system helps reduce the severity of pain. If this system is exhausted, the animal is left unprotected against distress and pain. This explains the out of proportion and painful response of RSD patients to any form of distress: a cold breeze, a family argument, or distress of alcohol withdrawal.

LIFE-THREATENING PAIN

Another dimension of quality of pain is the degree of arousal it causes in the central nervous system. Although there is a certain degree of overlap among acute pain, hyperpathic pain, and life-threatening pain, each of these dimensions is distinct and different.

The pain of an almost fatal heart attack disturbs the function of the CNS in a different fashion than the chest pain due to anxiety.

Sympathetic pain in the craniocervical region stimulates the brain stem through the trigeminal system more diffusely and has a more stressful and life-threatening effect on the CNS than the pain of acute appendicitis.

The pain of rape, with its life-threatening and shocking connotations, cannot even in the simplest and most superficial way be compared with the pain of rough "physical sex".

This third dimension of pain can make the difference between life and death, depending on the preexisting state of mind of the animal when inflicted with pain. A shark does not part with life as easily as a rabbit. A mother shows several times more resilience and power of survival if she has to get into a fight and sacrifice her life for her baby. A soldier hopeful for victory is more likely to survive a near-fatal battle.

This life-threatening dimension of pain not only can endow the patient with superhuman fighting power, but it can help the patient become more tolerant of the pain. In this regard it helps the survival of the species, but confuses the student of quality of pain.

It seems that chronic pain, especially causalgic chronic pain, is not conducive to emotional and physical stoicism. Suicide, stroke, and heart attack are more common among these patients.

This aspect of the pain is discussed below under the subject of stress and RSD.

ORIGINS OF SIA AND SIP

STRESS-INDUCED PAIN (SIP)

As briefly mentioned above and voluminously detailed in the medical literature, there are two different types of stress-induced pain.

What makes the two different is environmental circumstances such as war vs. peace or sex vs. rape type of stress, as well as the effect of painful stress on the body (eustress vs. distress).

Historically it has been well known that pain can be tolerated if it is accompanied by endorphin-stimulated exercises, e.g., dances of the Dervishes, which makes them tolerant of pain to the extent that the endorphin-generating exercises enable them to inflict holes in their tongues or faces.

We need to return to neurophysiology to find the answers for SIA.

The first report of SIA was by Akil et al.[462] in 1970. They induced SIA in rats that was neutralized by narcotic antagonists. The rats previously given naloxone did not achieve SIA. This proved **endorphins** and other **opioid peptides** are instrumental both in SIA and SIP.

On the other hand, Hayes et al.[463] in 1978 induced SIA that was not blocked by naloxone.

The works of Terman et al.[464] point to two anatomical and hormonal types of SIA. Terman demonstrated that the same common pain receptors are influenced differently — according to circumstances — by opioid or nonopioid SIA instigating chemicals.

CHEMICALS INFLUENCING STRESS-INDUCED ANALGESIA (SIA)

SIA is a part of **adaption** of the animal toward **stress**. This adaptation is exerted through the cortical-hypothalamic axis down through the sympathetic adrenal axis. This is essential for protection of the **immune system** as well as **cardiovascular systems**.[465]

The peptides, β-endorphins and ACTH, are simultaneously released after exposure to stress.[466] If the animal has undergone hypoplysectomy, then the SIA mechanism disappears.[467]

GABA also plays a major inhibitory role in the dorsal horn of the spinal cord to achieve SIA.

The peptides β-endorphin (see Chapter 7, endorphins) and GABA are instrumental in the descending inhibitory system of SIA: inhibiting the firing of lamina 1 of the dorsal horn of the spinal cord.[469] The monoamine serotonin exerts a similar effect.

Dynorphin is a strong pain inhibitor in the dorsal horn. Its effect lasts up to 4 days.

The peptide substance P (see Chapter 7, substance P) along with norepinephrine plays a major role in the afferent ascending excitatory circuit of SIA and SIP. The impulses start from layer 1 of the dorsal horn ascending to the brain stem.

Neurotensin, a 13 amino acid peptide, also acts as a pain inhibitor in the dorsal horn of the spinal cord.

At present it is not clear which kind of stress induces a nonopioid type of SIA.

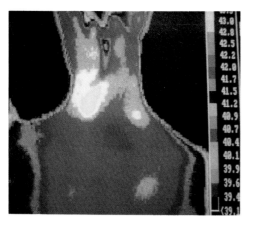

FIGURE 2a

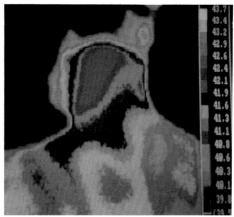

FIGURE 2b

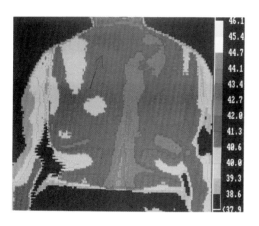

FIGURE 3

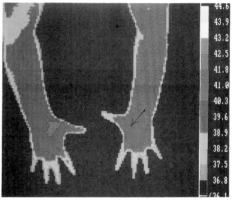

FIGURE 4b

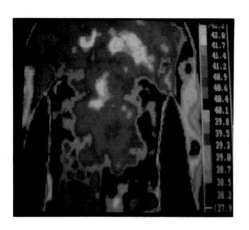

FIGURE 4d

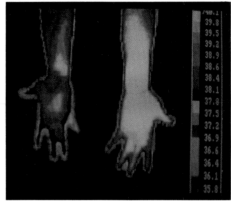

FIGURE 5a

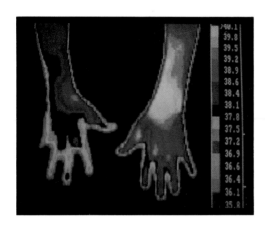

FIGURE 5b1

FIGURE 5b2

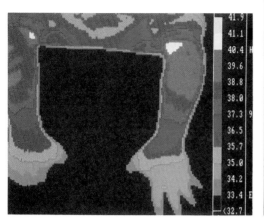

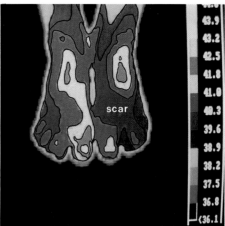

FIGURE 5c   FIGURE 6a

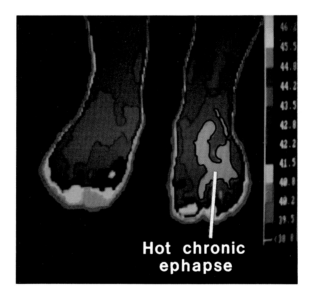

FIGURE 7

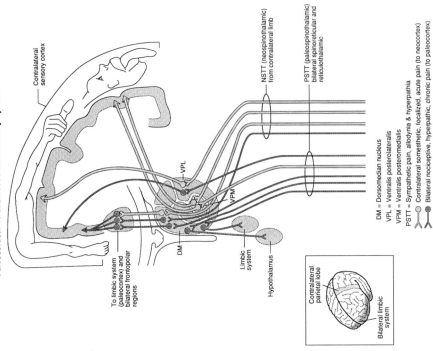

Paleocortical Versus Neocortical Sensory System

Contralateral sensory cortex

To limbic system (paleocortex) and bilateral frontopolar regions

VPL

VPM

DM

Limbic system

Hypothalamus

NSTT (neospinothalamic) from contralateral limb

PSTT (paleospinothalamic) bilateral spinoreticular and reticulothalamic

Contralateral parietal lobe

Bilateral limbic system

DM = Dorsomedian nucleus
VPL = Ventralis posterolateralis
VPM = Ventralis posteromedialis
PSTT = Sympathetic pain, allodynia & hyperpathia

Contralateral somesthetic, localized, acute pain (to neocortex)

Bilateral nociceptive, hyperpathic, chronic pain (to paleocortex)

FIGURE 12a

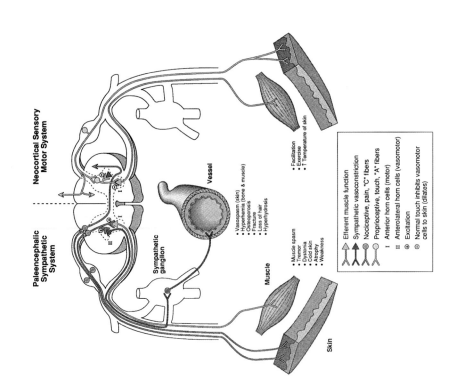

Neocortical Sensory Motor System

Paleencephalic Sympathetic System

Vessel

Sympathetic ganglion

Muscle

Skin

• Vasospasm (skin)
• Hyperhemia (bone & muscle)
• Osteoporosis
• Fracture
• Loss of hair
• Hyperhydrosis

• Muscle spasm
• Tremor
• Dystonia
• Cold skin
• Atrophy
• Weakness

• Facilitation
• Exercise
• ↑ Temperature of skin

Efferent muscle function
Sympathetic vasoconstriction
Nociceptive, pain, "C" fibers
Proprioceptive, touch, "A" fibers
I   Anterior horn cells (motor)
II   Anterolateral horn cells (vasomotor)
⊕   Excitation
⊖   Normal touch inhibits vasomotor cells to skin (dilates)

FIGURE 9

III. Peripheral Scar (Ephapse, Causalgia) RSD

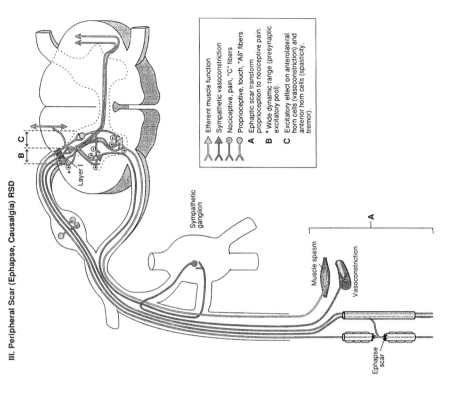

Efferent muscle function
Sympathetic vasoconstriction
Nociceptive, pain, "C" fibers
Proprioceptive, touch, "Aδ" fibers

A   Ephaptic scar transform
    proprioception to nociceptive pain.
B   *Wide dynamic range (presynaptic
    excitatory pool).
C   Excitatory effect on anterolateral
    horn cells (vasoconstriction) and
    anterior horn cells (spasticity,
    tremor).

Layer I

Sympathetic
ganglion

Muscle spasm

Vasoconstriction

Ephapse
scar

A

FIGURE 14

II. Disuse RSD (Inactivity) Due to Pain

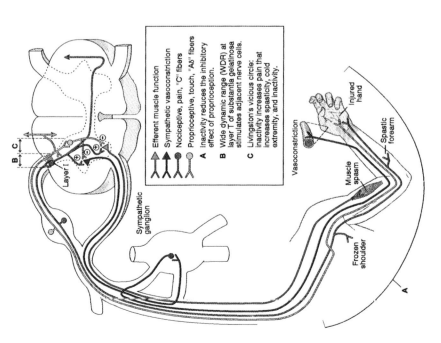

Efferent muscle function
Sympathetic vasoconstriction
Nociceptive, pain, "C" fibers
Proprioceptive, touch, "Aδ" fibers

A   Inactivity reduces the inhibitory
    effect of proprioception.
B   Wide dynamic range (WDR) at
    layer T of substantia gelatinosa
    stimulates adjacent nerve cells.
C   Livingston's vicious circle:
    inactivity increases pain that
    increases spasticity, cold
    extremity, and inactivity.

Layer I

Sympathetic
ganglion

Vasoconstriction

Muscle
spasm

Frozen
shoulder

Injured
hand

Spastic
forearm

A

FIGURE 13a

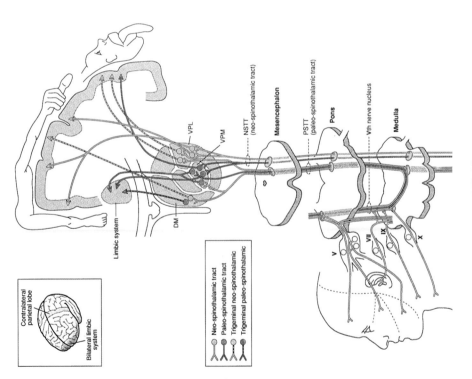

Referred Pain

Referred pain

Vth nerve

Scar soft tissue injury

Cervical sensory nerve roots

C1
C2
C3
C4

Substantia gelatinosa & trigeminal nucleus overlap

To shoulder (referred pain)

Sherrington's overlapping afferent pools

A B C

Cervical afferents
Trigeminal afferents

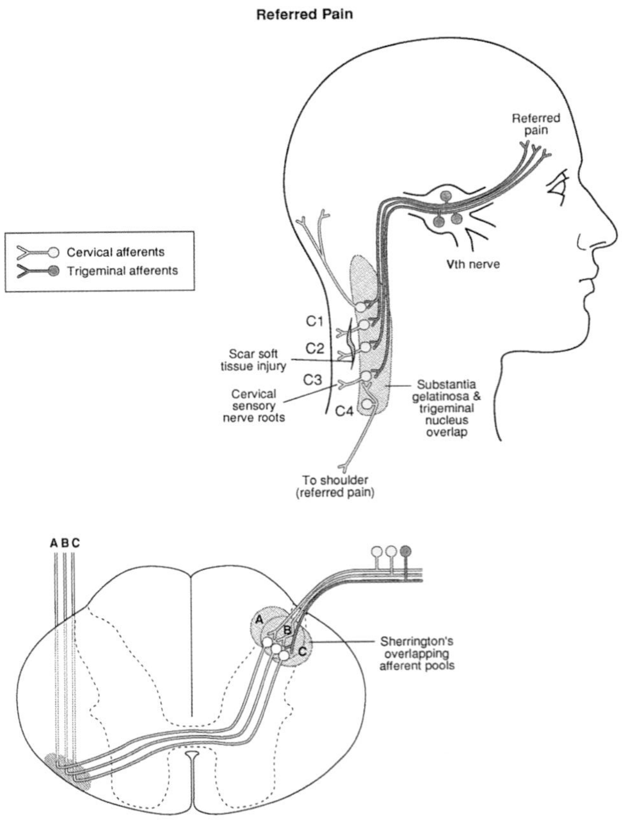

FIGURE 16

Contralateral parietal lobe

Bilateral limbic system

Limbic system

DM

VPL
VPM

NSTT (neo-spinothalamic tract)

Mesencephalon

PSTT (paleo-spinothalamic tract)

Pons

Vth nerve nucleus

Medulla

V
VII
IX
X

Neo-spinothalamic tract
Paleo-spinothalamic tract
Trigeminal neo-spinothalamic
Trigeminal paleo-spinothalamic

FIGURE 15

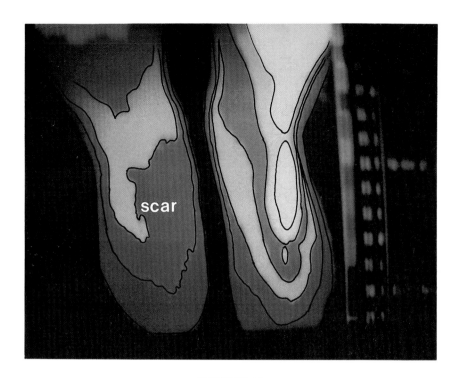

FIGURE 20

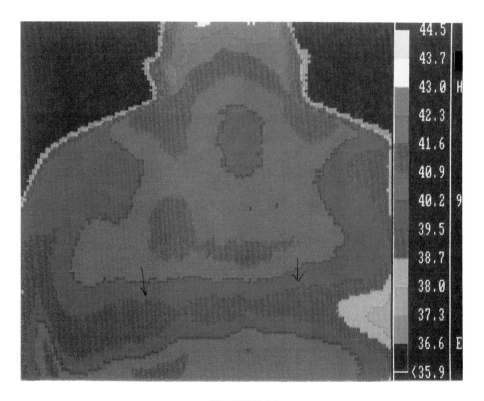

FIGURE 24

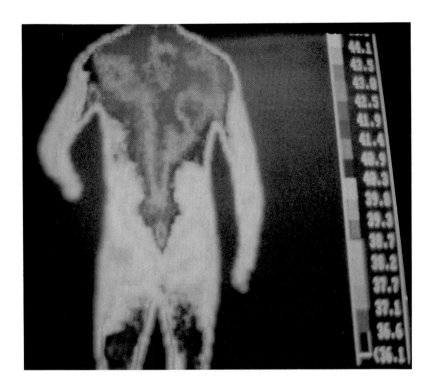

FIGURE 25

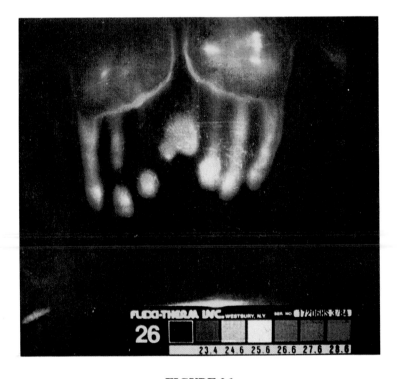

FIGURE 26

Studies by Duncan et al.[468] revealed that SIA can be turned on by anticipation long before the noxious stimulus is applied. The studies by Duncan et al.[468] revealed that the above-mentioned anticipation is influenced by contingent behavioral changes from RVM through thalamocortical connections of the frontal lobe. Ever since the early 1961 physiologic works of Greg Walters, the anticipatory role of the frontal lobe [called contingent negative variance or (CNV)] has been established.

It is concluded that pain is not always "bad" or harmful. **Pain is necessary** for proper function of the stress response and the immune system.

There are two types of pain: SIA-modulated pain as in acute pain and in normal **eustress**, and SIP-modulated pain as in **distress** and in **complex chronic pain** (CCP) (Figures 12a and 12b).

SYMPATHETIC MEDIATED PAIN (SMP)

Sympathetic pain, also known as **hyperpathic, allodynic,** or **neuropathic pain,** is different from somatic or somesthetic pain due to the fact that the pain is out of proportion to the peripheral injury, and it is accompanied by a burning feeling (allodynia) that is quite disabling and intolerable (hyperpathia). The pain impulse is transferred through the c fibers.

The afferent painful stimuli persist and perpetuate in the internuncial pool of the spinal cord, which in turn exaggerates and increases the afferent and efferent sympathetic activity (wide dynamic range).[242]

SOMESTHETIC (SOMATIC) PAIN VS. SYMPATHETIC PAIN (SMP)

The two pain systems (Table 5) have been recognized as two independent structures as early as the 1960s by the late Dr. Kerr,[580] my professor of neurosurgery at the Mayo Clinic. Only in the past 5 to 6 years has the existence of an old limbic pain system as contrasted with a laterally positioned somesthetic pain system (starting from the lateral spinothalamic tract and ending in the contralateral parietal lobe) been generally recognized and accepted by algologists.

Pain is an integral part of normal physiologic sensation. It is a defense mechanism that is absolutely necessary. RSD in itself is a hyperpathic pain. It is a typical chronic pain, and chronic pain is the best example of pathologic pain.

Microneurography[124,385] and intraneural microstimulation[252,253,373] experiments reveal that pain can be elicited in human beings when either A fibers or C nociceptor units are activated. The physiologic pain by such experiments can be divided into the following:

1. Sharp pain, which is activated by A-δ nociceptors.
2. Dull pain due to activation of C-nociceptors.
3. Cramp type of pain, which is usually more of a referred pain rather than being due to single stimulation of either the A or c fibers.[252,373,374]

Naturally, the physiologic type of pain is transient, quite focalized, and usually disappears without any significant residual. It can cause transient changes in vital signs (pulse, blood pressure, etc.).

MANIFESTATION OF SYMPATHETIC (HYPERPATHIC) PAIN

Pathologic pain has a variety of manifestations such as **neuropathic, hyperpathic,** and **allodynic** (burning) pain of RSD. There are unlimited types of pathologic pain, as the different examples mentioned above are seen in combination or in different severity and duration. The pathologic pain quite frequently results in referred pain. The referred pain explains the complexity of the pathologic pain and its distribution. It explains how acupuncture alleviates the pain. Acupuncture stimulates the larger A-δ fibers, and the overlap of the A-δ fiber stimulation with the c fiber stimulation of hyperpathic pain results in a masking of the c fiber type of pain and temporary relief of pain. Its best use is in the form of anesthesia. Acupuncture is useless for treatment of chronic pain because of its temporary effect. While the patient undergoes acupuncture, the pain is relieved, only to recur a few hours later.

Sympathetic pain is not a discrete focalized pain, but has a **tendency to spread** to adjacent neural structures. This fact causes confusion in diagnosis. The spread of pain from hand to shoulder results in the shoulder-hand syndrome. Pain around the shoulder area may be misdiagnosed as bursitis or rotator cuff injury. The spread of pain from the cervical spine to the craniofacial structures is commonly misdiagnosed as migraine or trigeminal neuralgia.

ORIGINS OF SYMPATHETIC PAIN

(1) RSD OF DISUSE (Figure 5d)

Sympathetic pain originates from an injury that affects the c fibers. It has two major origins:

(1) **inactivity (RSD of disuse)** that results in reduction of proprioception (touch and position), and
(2) secondary lack of inhibition of anterolateral horn cells.

This results in vasoconstriction and cold extremity with secondary further reduction of proprioception and hyperactivity of anterolateral horn cells (Figures 11, 13, and 14).

RSD frequently is the result of an injury causing pain with secondary inactivity (RSD of disuse).

> RSD of Disuse = Inactivity → Reduced Proprioception
> → Uninhibited Anterolateral Horn Cells
> → Vasoconstriction → Reduced Proprioception
> → Repetition of Vicious Circle (Figures 11 and 13)

(2) SCAR (EPHAPTIC) PAIN

When pathologic pain has a peripheral origin in the form of scar formation (Figures 5–8 and 14), the damaged c fibers in the area of injury are capable of engaging in spontaneous and **nonspecific mechanosensitive ectopic discharges** with resultant **ephaptic** (in contrast to synaptic) **cross-talk**.[33]

Experiments by Blumberg and Janig[33] have demonstrated that electrical cross-talk can be the source of pathologic pain. Granit et al.,[118] Seitzer and Devor,[334] and Rasminsky[289–291] have clearly exemplified the ephapse or cross-talk in the scarred nerve fibers both in the skin (Figure 8) as well as in the sensory nerve roots (Figures 8 and 14). The ephaptic cross-talk results in major and minor causalgias. The ephaptic response can activate sensory as well as motor nerve fibers (Figures 11, 13, and 14). The best examples of motor nerve fiber in ephaptic response are vasoconstriction, spasticity, tremor, and hemifacial spasm.[245–247]

Another practical clinical example of ephaptic transfer is nerve root contusion (Table 7, Chapter 6) and partial nerve root avulsion, which are quite frequently accompanied by spontaneous pathologic hyperpathic pain and RSD.[424]

In this type of nerve root contusion (Table 7) or avulsion pain, the ephaptic source of pain may be due to partial disruption of the nerve root or may be due to total avulsion with the central end of the avulsed nerve being the source of ephaptic pain and acting similar to stump phantom pain.

DEAFFERENTATION

In all different forms of ephaptic pain, be it in the skin, peripheral nerves (Figures 8 and 14) or in the nerve roots, or even in the spinal cord, deafferentation results in spontaneous pathologic input of painful impulse. **Deafferentation** refers to the lack of inhibitory influence on anterolateral and anterior horn cells by A-δ fibers.

The deafferentation after injury to the nociceptor fibers in the spinal canal can cause **spontaneous electrical discharges**. Such a phenomenon is noted in patients with **partial spinal cord injury**, which can result in attacks of **myoclonic** or **akinetic seizure** involving the lower extremities. The epileptiform focus obviously cannot be recorded on scalp EEG

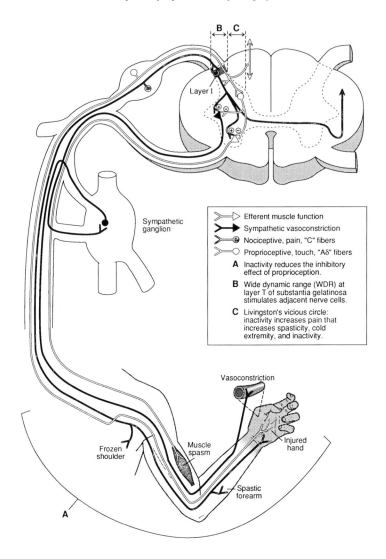

FIGURE 13a. RSD of disuse. Note A, B, and C on diagram: (A) Peripherally, inactivity due to pain reduces proprioceptive input and its inhibitory effect on the anterolateral horn cells of the spinal cord. (B) The uninhibited pain input at layer 1 of substantia gelatinosa stimulates the adjacent nerve cells (wide dynamic range or WDR effect). (C) At the anterolateral horn cells level the reduced proprioceptive input leaves the sympathetic output uninhibited (Livingston's vicious circle). See also color plates following page 42.

recording. However, somatosensory evoked potential (SSEP) recording of the spinal cord function is invariably abnormal in such patients. This is especially true in electrical injuries (see Electrical Injuries, and Figure 25).

The spinal cord (Figures 8, 9, and 11) plays a major role in **allodynia** (burning pain).[242,300,362,363] The pathologic pain of deafferentation is usually accompanied by autonomic manifestations of RSD. One example of such autonomic manifestation is **idiopathic hyperhydrosis**. With this congenital illness, just simple touch and mechanoreceptor type of stimulus result in **excessive reflex sweating bilaterally in the extremities**. This phenomenon in a partial fashion is seen in most chronic forms of RSD.

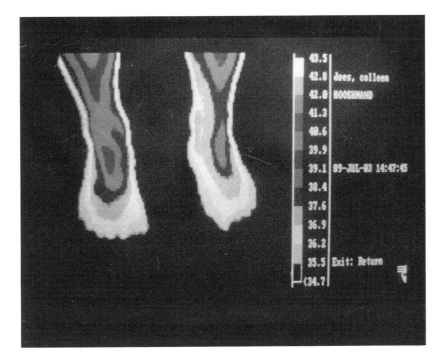

FIGURE 13b. Concentric reduction of peripheral temperature in distal thermatomes of the extremity due to RSD of disuse involving left foot. There is no thermatomal disruption.

The large somatic proprioceptive fibers transmit position and vibration sense. Pain is transmitted through the c fibers. Peripheral injury with scar formation results in a crossover (electric short) between these two systems (Figures 8 and 14). As a result, the pain impulses are shorted from c fibers to large proprioceptive fibers.[393] This in turn augments the feeling of pain by causing painful paresthesias.

The **scar formation** disrupts the insulating effect of myelin, and it causes an **electric short** between the adjacent large and small fibers (Figure 14). As a result, recruitment and exaggeration of pain impulse develop in the area of scar (ephaptic pain).

The **ephaptic** transmission results in a **crossover of sensory (afferent) impulses to vasomotor (efferent) fibers** (Figure 14) distal to the area of the scar with secondary **exaggerated vasoconstriction** typical of ephaptic reflex sympathetic dystrophy.[186]

The increased activity in the **internuncial pools** in the spinal cord or brain results in stimulation of more than one level of the spinal cord.[196,242,301] As a result, the **CNS is stimulated out of proportion** and interprets even the smallest source of RSD pain as a diffused stimulation of the CNS with **secondary exaggerated pain out of proportion** to the original stimulus.

The resultant **allodynia** (burning pain) and **hyperpathia** (exaggerated pain) are on the basis of diffused stimulation of the spinal cord and on the basis of peripheral mechanoreceptor discharge of the c fibers, causing **repetitive hyperactivity** of the efferent sympathetic nervous system with resultant **vicious circle of Livingston**.[196,301]

Normally, the opposing inhibitory effects of proprioceptive (position) vs. excitatory effect of nociceptive (pain) fibers on the anterolateral horn cells of the spinal cord result in a steady state of isothermic heat loss in the skin of the extremities. The **perpetuating injurious ephaptic pain** tilts the balance toward excitation of the anterolateral horn cells resulting in vasoconstriction.

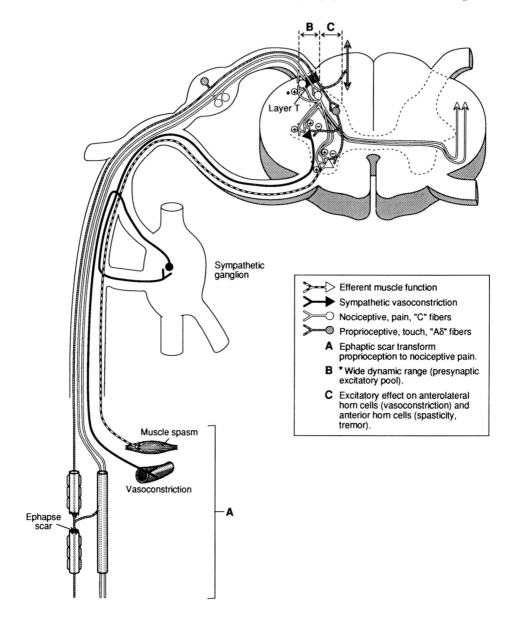

FIGURE 14. Ephaptic RSD: peripheral nerve damage causes disruption of insulating protection of myelin sheath. This causes ephapse (cross-stimulation of adjacent nerve fibers, in contrast to selective, insulated synaptic stimulation). As a result, a simple touch can cause stimulation of sensory pain fibers. The ephaptic sensory stimulation causes exaggerated sympathetic stimulation (causalgia). See also color plates following page 42.

The resultant inactivity (Figure 13) due to the severity of the pain causes **lack of inhibitory effect of proprioceptive input** on the anterolateral horn cells of the spinal cord, and secondarily results in unopposed (Figures 13 and 14) **hyperactivity of the sympathetic vasoconstriction.**[197]

The augmentation and recruitment of the pain input is further exaggerated by the angry backfiring c fibers (ABC of OCHOA)[249] in the periphery. This is true only when there is damage to adjacent sensory fibers in the periphery (Figure 8 and 14), resulting in electric short (**ephapse**) in the adjacent c fibers.

CENTRAL TRANSMISSION OF SYMPATHETIC PAIN

The **sympathetic pain**, phylogenetically a **more primitive** and **hyperpathic pain** (Figures 10 and 13), follows a **different route in CNS (medial pain system)** than the more sophisticated somatic pain (lateral pain system). The c fibers carrying nociceptive afferent impulses end up in layer 1 (superficial layer) (Figures 11, 13, and 14) of the posterior horn of the spinal cord. From there (Figures 11b, 13b, and 14b) they stimulate a wide dynamic range[415,416] of adjacent levels of the spinal cord, resulting in a diffuse nociceptive pain. They eventually end up in the prefrontal cortex, inducing anxiety (Figure 12). This is in contrast with the A-δ fibers, which end up in the deeper layers of the posterior horn and relay to the lateral spinothalamic tract. The pain transmission in this tract is a discrete focalized pain that ends up in the sensory cortex of the contralateral parietal lobe, and it is not accompanied by hyperpathia and its emotional connotations (Table 5).

The lateral spinothalamic (neospinothalamic or NSTT) carries the discrete somatic type of impulse. In contrast, the pain impulse mainly responsible for RSD travels mostly through the paleospinothalamic tract (PSTT) and to a lesser extent through the neospinothalamic tract (NSTT) (Figure 12).

The main difference between the paleospinothalamic vs. the neospinothalamic tract is not only phylogenetic but also anatomical.

The lateral spinothalamic tract (LSTT), which is mainly responsible for somatic pain, terminates in the ventralis posterolateralis (VPL) nuclei of the thalamus where the fibers synapse with neurons that provide input to the neurosensory cortex in a discrete somatotypically organized fashion (Figure 12).

As a result, these fibers transmit clear-cut discrete feeling from circumscribed areas of the body to the neocortex.

In contrast, the paleospinothalamic fibers take the path of the spinoreticular and spinomesencephalic tract (SRT and SMT). They are multisynaptic, diffuse in their projection, and stimulate the reticular formation at the periaqueductal gray (PAG), the hypothalamus (H), nucleus submedium, and medial intralaminar dynamic nuclei of the thalamus (MIT) (Figure 12).

Eventually these fibers stimulate the limbic forebrain system causing a feeling of hyperpathia, allodynia, unpleasant pain, and exacerbated and augmented pain. This type of pain involves the paleocortex and is quite diffuse with a strong emotional connotation in contrast to the neospinothalamic type of pain. It has ipsilateral as well as contralateral projections to the frontal lobe with resultant emotional alarm (hyperpathia) and severe anxiety. The ipsilateral projections terminate in the mesial frontal lobe regions with resultant anxiety, hypertension, insomnia, and secondary depression (Figures 12a and 15).

SUMMARY

As the nociceptive impulses of autonomic pain enter the spinal cord, they end up in PSTT cells of origin, which are in the deeper laminae of the posterior horn of the spinal cord. They ascend in the deeper portion of the spinothalamic tract, have multiple relays in the reticular formation of the brain stem, and follow the tract in the periaqueductal gray up to the hypothalamus, medialis dorsalis, and intralaminar thalamic nuclei.

They synapse with neurons that connect with the limbic forebrain system (Figures 12 and 21) with resultant stimulation of the complex circuits in the entire limbic system: paleocortex in temporal lobe as well as mesial frontal lobe regions. The stimulation of the limbic system results in distress (fight or flight) reaction as well as depression, and the frontal lobe stimulation results in anxiety, hypertension, panic, and tachycardia.

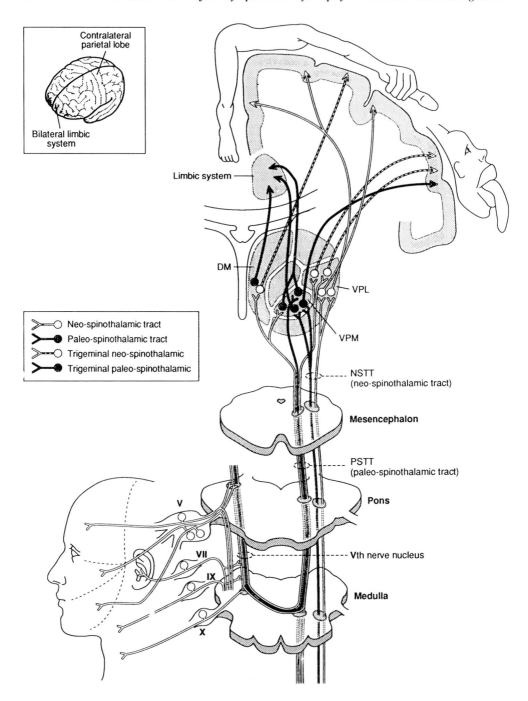

FIGURE 15. The trigeminal nervous system is comprised of paleo- and neospinothalamic anatomical structures.[580] As a result, craniocervical injuries are likely to undergo RSD. See also color plates following page 42.

CLINICAL EXAMPLES OF PALEENCEPHALIC (SYMPATHETIC) PAIN
The following are some clinical examples of paleencephalic vs. neospinothalamic pain:

1. Transcutaneous nerve stimulator (TNS) is an excellent example of neospinothalamic transmission. Repetitive electrical stimulation by TNS through the small and large pain fibers blocks off the input of paleencephalic c fiber type of pain and stimulates the cerebral cortical inhibitory gray matter, which in turn inhibits paleencephalic unpleasant pain.

2. In patients who have suffered from head injury and are in a coma, simple touch or checking reflexes may not cause any significant arousal. However, on the same patients, stimulation of c fibers by using a cotton swab and stimulating the nasal hair cause a significant arousal response through the interlaminar granular cells of the thalamus (Figure 12). This is nothing but a wide dynamic range phenomenon at the brain stem and thalamic levels (Figure 15).

    In the above example of stimulating the nasal hair in a comatose patient with resultant marked arousal, the c fibers of the nasal hair region stimulate the reticular thalamic fibers in a diffuse fashion with base of arousal being in the paleencephalic areas of the thalamic cortical distribution.

3. Surgical scars, due to treatment of acute surgical emergencies or elective surgical procedures, heal nicely in a few days or weeks without any further complications. However, entrapment of a peripheral nerve or formation of a neuroma at the scar region or in an amputated stump changes the temporary somesthetic pain to a hyperpathic pain that never stops.

4. In patients who have suffered from facial bone fracture and have developed a migraine vascular type of headache, ingestion of ice water or ice cream can be a trigger point mechanism and starts a severe migraine vascular headache. The same patients may get relief from TNS or a modified form of TNS called *pain suppressor*, which stimulates larger neospinothalamic type of nerve fibers (neocortical stimulation).

5. The paleencephalic stimulation is more likely to occur in craniocervical region injuries. The craniocervical afferent fibers have an extensive overlap with the reticular system of the brain stem (Figure 15). This results in Sherrington's phenomenon[573] (Figure 16). As a result, the reticulothalamocortical fibers are stimulated more easily than when there is an afferent stimulation from the rest of the body. The same principle explains the frequent complication of posttraumatic vascular migrainous types of headache after cranial, facial, and cervical injuries (Figures 16, 18a, and 18b).

MODULATORS OF PALEOSPINOTHALAMIC TRACT

Sleep has an inhibitory effect on the PSTT system, whereas stimulants, arousal, anger, hostility, and depression cause a lowered threshold for this PSTT (paleospinothalamic pain system). Narcotics, alcohol, and benzodiazepines temporarily suppress this system. Withdrawal from these addicting drugs causes a significant augmentation of the emotional connotations of PSTT pain (Figure 19).

The neocortex has a modulatory effect on the PSTT system with positive and negative two-way feedback.

The granular cells of the frontal lobe neocortex exert an inhibitory effect on this system. The pyramidal cells have the opposite effect. The more immature and the more uninhibited the frontal lobe, the more uninhibited is the PSTT system.

The best example of this poor inhibition of the frontal lobe is the more prominent clinical picture of **RSD among children** and among the people of more primitive cultures. The more

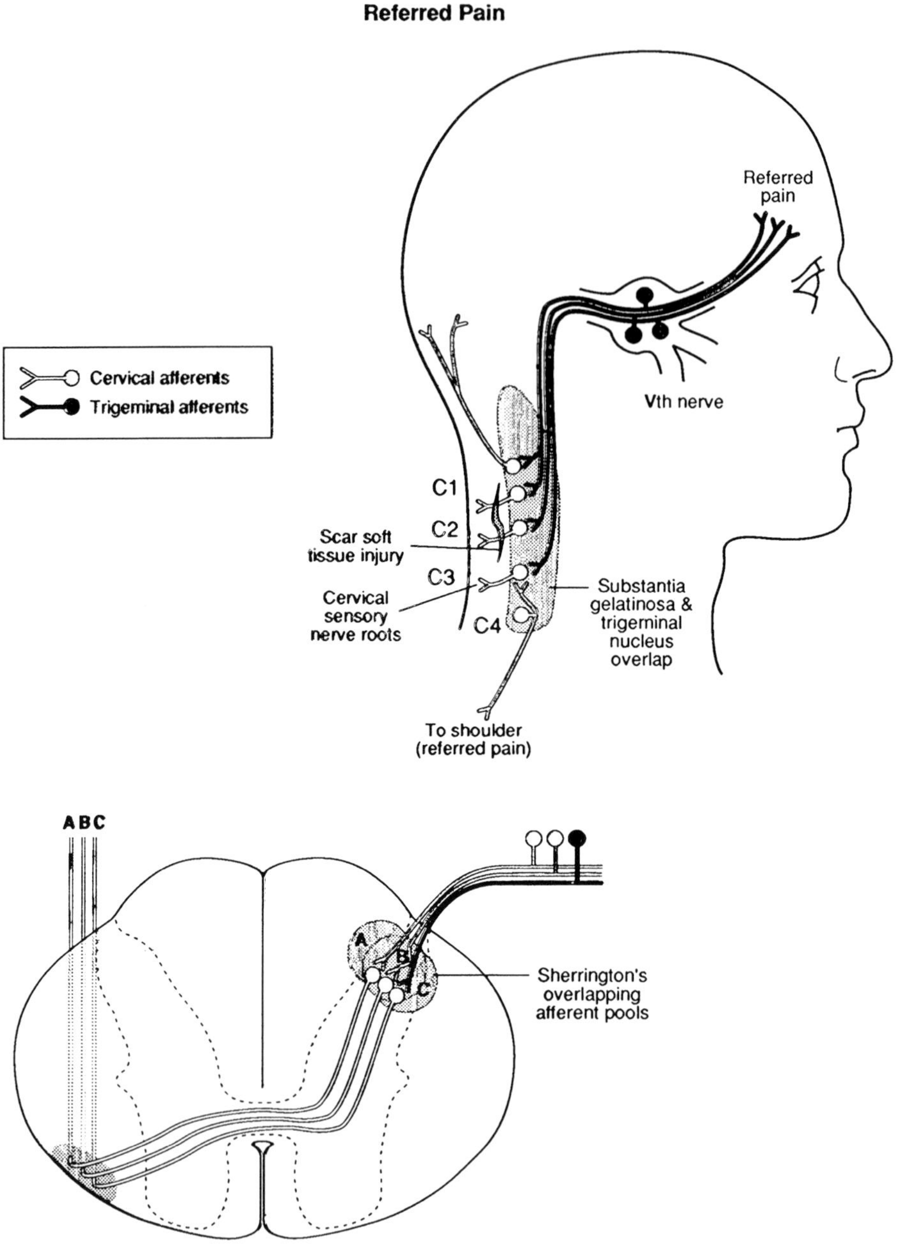

Referred Pain

FIGURE 16. Sherrington[579] and Kerr[580] phenonmenon points to the overlapping afferent sensory pools. This results in spread of sensory input to adjacent areas of substantia gelatinosa and the phenomenon of referred pain. The pain of appendicitis may be felt in the epigastric region. The pain due to soft injuries to the cervical spine region may be referred to the shoulder and arm or the ophthalmic branch of the trigeminal nerve, causing frontal and retroorbital headache, typical of migraine. See also color plates following page 42.

primitive the culture, the less understanding they have of the dynamics of pain. The more emphasis on social superstition, the more exaggerated is the effect of RSD. The same is true in patients who basically have neurotic histrionic personalities.

There has been a proper emphasis in the literature in regard to the exacerbation of RSD in **younger children**.[13,63,187,323,339] In children and adolescents, RSD is accompanied by a more

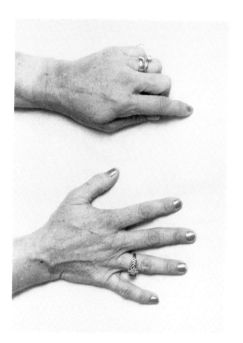
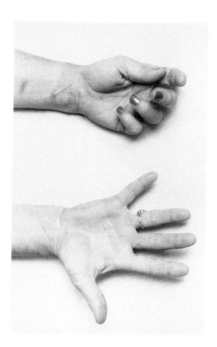

FIGURE 17. Mild left C7 and C8 nerve roots contusion and secondary RSD and flexion deformity diagnosed as and operated on with no success: (a) tardy ulnar palsy; (b) ulnar nerve entrapment at the wrist; (c) carpal tunnel syndrome; (d) thoracic outlet syndrome. Treatment with regional block, physiotherapy, and carisoprodol resulted in muscle relaxation and useful hand.

severe pain, bone loss, and **muscular weakness.** The clinical picture is more impressive than the same in adults;[187,337] yet, the **prognosis is better** than in adults probably due to the **surge of hormones in the second decade of life.**

The same is true in the trigeminal distribution type of RSD, which results in vascular (migrainous) headaches after head injury. This condition is **more severe in children.**

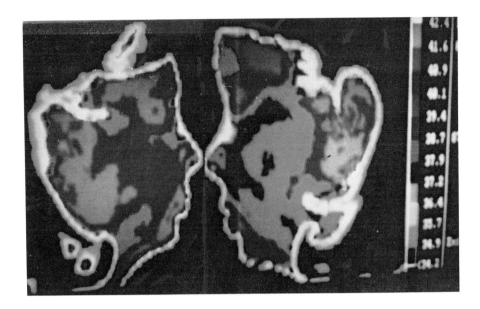

FIGURE 18a. Left cervical spine injury with left-sided severe headache and left Horner's syndrome[581] diagnosed as *cluster headache*. Treatment with prednisolone, sansert, and other standard medications for cluster headache failed. Physiotherapy to cervical spine, trigger point injection, TNS, along with treatment with stellate block and Verapamil controlled the headache and face pain. Thermography showed cold spot left C3 cervical paraspinal region (treated with trigger point injection) as well as hypothermia in the distribution of left trigeminal nerve.

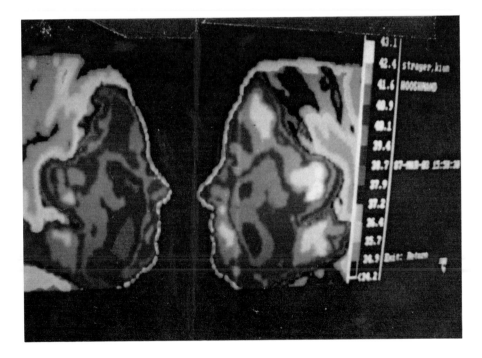

FIGURE 18b. Posttraumatic facial pain and RSD. Head and face injury (12 years earlier) with secondary headache and trigeminal neuralgia type of pain. Carbamazepine did not help. Treatment with Terazocin (α I blocker), physiotherapy, and pain suppressor stimulation (similar to TNS) resulted in excellent relief. Thermography was the only abnormal test.

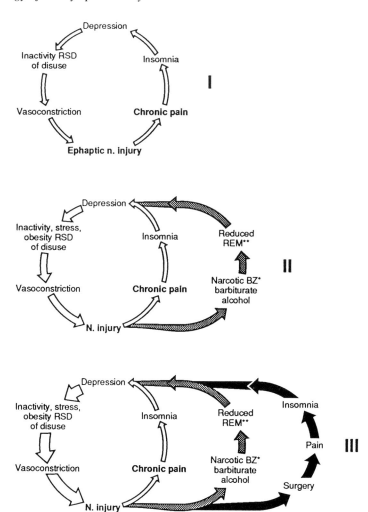

* BZ = Benzodiazepines (eg. valium, xanax, halcion)
** REM = Rapid eye movement sleep

FIGURE 19. Aggravation and perpetuation of chronic pain (RSD) by standard medications. Iatrogenic medicine is responsible for perpetuation of chronic pain in over 12 million people in the United States. The figure was extrapolated by applying the percentage of detoxification patients to the general population. Discontinuation of narcotics and sleeping pills (benzodiazepines) is the first step in management of chronic pain (especially RSD).

5
Sympathetic Nervous System and Motor Function

The sympathetic nervous system (SNS) not only modulates the nociceptive pain, but it also influences the efferent (motor) function.

1.   SNS controls vasoconstriction and provides control of circulation of organs.
2.   SNS controls the tonus of muscles. Excessive efferent output of SNS can result in **tremor** and **flexion deformity** of the extremity (Yokota et al.[425]) as well as **self-mutilating** behavior in animals.[6]
3.   The **selective therapeutic efficacy** of sympathetic proximal nerve block in relief of hyperpathic pain as opposed to nonhyperpathic pain[421] reflects the importance of **efferent pathways** in the development of RSD and hyperpathia.
4.   In causalgia, ephaptic electrical discharges cause **vasomotor** and **sudomotor hyperactivity, tremor, spasticity**, and **flexion deformity reflex**. The efferent portion of the SNS reflex arc is the originator of the above responses.[192,229,314]
5.   Clinically the efferent pathology of RSD has to be corrected to ensure success in treatment. This consists of sympathetic block, biofeedback, TNS, traction, and muscle relaxants, to name a few.

The following is an explanation of efferent function of SNS.

The **proprioceptive** (touch, position, and vibration) system exerts an **inhibitory effect** on the anterior horn cells (muscle relaxation) and anterolateral horn cells (reduction of sympathetic hyperactivity) (Figures 10, 11, 13, and 14).

On the other hand, the persistent input of **nociceptive sympathetic impulses** from the scarred area of the skin (ephaptic RSD) causes hyperactivity of the sympathetic nervous system, a persistent **vasoconstriction**, and **hypoxia** with perpetuation of pain as a **vicious circle** (Figure 13). It also causes contraction of muscles of the extremities through stimulation of anterior horn cells resulting in **spasm, tremor**, and even **dystonic movements** (Figures 10, 13, and 14).

The **sympathetic-originated spasm** involving facial muscles results in **TMJ disease**.

The same type of spasm involving scalenus muscles results in **thoracic outlet syndrome**.

Surgery in the case of TMJ disease or thoracic outlet syndrome results in vicious circle and aggravation of RSD. Hence, the importance of **muscle relaxants** in the treatment of RSD.

This muscle contraction causes further secretion of **lactic acid**, substance P, with secondary perpetuation of pain as a vicious circle.

Sympathetic block relieves **muscle contraction** and improves motor function of the extremity involved in RSD.[111–117] This muscle contraction can cause **vasospasms, involuntary movements, tremors** of different frequencies, **weakness,** and **dystonia,** which can be quite disabling.[112–117] It typically causes **flexion** deformity of **shoulder, elbow,** and **wrist** (Figures 13 and 14) and **hyperextension** deformity of the **knee.**

The two opposing sensory systems (proprioceptive vs. nociceptive) have an opposite influence in the tone and movement of the extremity. The **proprioceptive** (pleasant touch and exercise) impulse results in **facilitation of muscle activity, relaxation,** and **warming of the skin.**

On the other hand, the unpleasant **nociceptive** (sympathetic) impulse results in **hypertonicity, flexor muscles stimulation, spasticity, withdrawal, tremor, dystonia,** and cold skin.

TREATMENT APPLICATIONS

Recognition of the influence of the sympathetic nervous system on muscle function is quite essential in successful management of RSD. Medications such as **baclofen** (Lioresol) and carisoprodol (Soma) can be quite helpful in the management of the above-mentioned movement disorders.

The use of **sympathetic block, heat, biofeedback,** and **transcutaneous nerve stimulator** (TNS) on trigger points (but not on the area of scar) relieves the pain and movement disorder.

In contrast, the use of ice, TNS, and even simple touch on the ephaptic nerve-damaged scar has the opposite effect by causing increased nociceptive impulses and aggravation of ephaptic RSD.

6

Manifestations of RSD

RSD manifests itself in two main forms: (1) RSD of disuse and (2) RSD secondary to scar formation of peripheral nerves or ephaptic RSD: minor or major causalgia (Table 6).

Trauma is not the most common cause of RSD (see etiology). There are many forms of trauma:

1. Blunt trauma (more likely to cause disuse RSD)
2. Laceration over watershed zones (ephaptic RSD)
3. Bullet injuries (ephaptic: causalgic)
4. Electrocution (causalgic and disuse combination)
5. Sword or sharp knife injury (ephaptic injury)
6. Vibratory damage
    a. Drilling steel against titanium (disuse)
    b. Vibration of bullet injury

Locations of injury in the watershed areas include

1. Craniocervical (trigeminocervical watershed)
2. Dorsum of hand (radial-ulnar-median watershed)
3. Dorsum of foot (sural-superficial peroneal-deep peroneal watershed)
4. Anterolateral aspect of the knee
5. Palmar aspect of the wrist (median-ulnar watershed)

RSD OF DISUSE

The main function of the sympathetic nervous system is to provide proper circulation to the end organs according to demand. If an extremity is inactive, it is going to need less arterial blood — hence, vasoconstriction. The reverse is true with activity.

The mechanism of this proper and physiological sympathetic reflex is based on the principle of proprioception. Proprioception is the sensory input from the end organ to the CNS. The input of proprioception results in inhibition of activity of the anterolateral (intermediolateral) horn cells of the spinal cord, which is responsible for generation of vasoconstriction and sympathetic dystrophy. Less activity in the extremity results in less proprioceptive input to the CNS.

Reduction in activity of an arm results in proportionate reduction of proprioception from the extremity to the anterolateral horn cells of the spinal cord. Secondarily, as the proprioceptive inhibition of the anterolateral horn cells is decreased, these cells become uninhibited and cause vasoconstriction in the extremity (Figures 5d and 13b).

TABLE 6
RSD Types among 482 Consecutive Patients
Suffering from Chronic Pain and RSD
Followed for Over 5 Years[a]

RSD of disuse	82
Ephaptic RSD	19
	101 Total
Minor causalgia	11
Major causalgia	8

[a] To determine the incidence without thermography, the figure should be approximately divided by four.

The commonest form of RSD, RSD of disuse, is simply due to the vicious circle of inactivity perpetuating the sympathetic hyperactivity and pain of the original injury.

Usually the cause of this RSD is a blunt injury to an extremity. In the first few days, the injured extremity has a tendency to be inflamed with increased temperature due to soft tissue damage.

However, in a matter of a few days, substance P, lactic acid, and superoxide byproducts are usually absorbed, and the temperature of the extremity turns cold. If the soft tissue injury is severe enough, it is accompanied by emotional connotations of severe pain and by improper immobilization of the extremity, and the pain persists.

The lack of proprioceptive input changes the pain to hyperpathia, and secondary sympathetic vasoconstriction develops. At this point, the major painful input from the extremity dominates the path of the paleospinothalamic tract and results in the patient's subconscious guarding of the extremity. This secondary inactivity aggravates sympathetic vasoconstriction and starts the vicious circle of disuse RSD.

Vasoconstriction results in secondary hypoxic irritation of the C fibers in the extremity and aggravation of pain. The secondary pain causes more inactivity, and thus results in more decreased circulation. The vicious circle eventually causes intractable pain.

Microneurographic recordings have linked the reverse relationship between the electrical activity of mechanoreceptor (Pacinian corpuscles and muscle spindles) and bursts of activity in sympathetic efferent fibers.[397]

The inactivity also results in development of bursitis and calcium formation around the tendons and around the shoulder or hip, and that in turn causes secondary pain that aggravates and exacerbates the vicious circle. The resultant frozen shoulder has its referred-pain origin in substantia gelatinosa of the cervical spinal cord (Figure 16).

In turn, unnecessary bracing or unnecessary application of a cast to the extremity perpetuates the vicious circle and magnifies RSD.

This mechanism of development of RSD results in improper diagnoses such as rotator cuff syndrome, bursitis, or shoulder, elbow, or hip sprain with secondary inactivity and aggravation of the condition.

EPHAPTIC (CAUSALGIC) RSD

In the less common form of RSD called ephaptic RSD (minor and major causalgias) not only is inactivity a problem, but also injury to the C fibers in the extremity or in the face results in ephaptic dystrophy.

Ephapse is defined as an **artifical synapse**, which by virtue of electrical transmission through two adjacent denuded and scarred nerves causes an electrical short. This electrical

TABLE 7
Causes of Neck and Back Pain in 482 Patients
with Detailed Studies[a]

Cause of pain	Number	Percent
Sympathetic dystrophy	101[b]	21.0[c]
Disc protrusion	135	28.0
Nerve roots contusion	94	22.0
Conversion reaction	66	15.4
Myofascial injuries	42	9.8
Electrical injuries	32	7.5
Arachnoiditis	12	2.8
Referred pain[d]	6[d]	1.4
Lumbar stenosis	16	3.7
Spinal cord injury	4	1.0
Total	508[e]	119.8%[e]

[a] EMG, SSEP, thermography as well as CT or MRI.
[b] Sympathetic dystrophy may have been alone or accompanied with other causes of the patient's pain. This accounts for the value of 508 and 119.8%.
[c] The RSD was diagnosed with the help of thermography. Divide the figures by 4 for incidence of RSD without thermography.
[d] Cancer, aortic aneurysm, pelvic injury.
[e] Multiple pathologies in a patient caused the total numbers and total percents to exceed the actual number of patients.

shunting bypasses the normal synaptic cleft and results in excitation of multiple nerve fibers (Figure 14). It may be due to demyelination (e.g., diabetes) or trauma. It causes pain and muscle weakness. EMG may show coupling discharges in distal muscles. In rare cases the same phenomenon has been reported in normal monkey peripheral nerves.[380] However, it is not clear if the normal monkey that shows coupling discharges on neurophysiologic test secondary to ephaptic conduction is truly "normal" or not. At least in human beings, this kind of coupling discharge is invariably pathological.

The ephapse in the peripheral nerve causes shunting of the electrical current from the C fibers (afferent ephaptic C fibers) to somatic afferent fibers (Figure 14) at the area of the scar.[381–386] The same ephaptic cross-talk has been demonstrated in primate experiments both in ephapse in the trunk of the nerve as well as in regenerating neuroma.[387–389]

Whereas standard forms of RSD are seen in approximately one third of chronic pain patients (Tables 6, 7, and 42), the classic major causalgia is seen in less than 5% of such patients.[374]

The old theory of the requirement of a penetrating missile wound does not hold any longer, and other forms of less severe trauma can cause major causalgia.[376–379] However, sharp objects and vibration due to drilling or secondary to missile and bullet velocity are the main contributors to major causalgia.

Injuries such as surgical scar, motorcycle and other vehicular avulsions of the peripheral nerves or brachial plexus, and in rare cases i.v. injection injury[376] are some of the usual civil causes of major causalgia.

NERVE ROOT CONTUSION (EPHAPTIC)

Contusion (Table 7) of sciatic nerve branches is responsible for around 40% of major causalgias. Median nerve is the second most common nerve involved (35%), followed by brachial plexus (12%) and by other less frequently involved nerves.[363,368,374]

Other nerves that are quite commonly involved in up to 10% of the patients consist of contusion of the ulnar nerve at the elbow and trigeminal nerve branches injury over the scalp or face.

The same phenomenon has been reported in animals suffering from axonal damage and demyelination.[389–391] Posttraumatic demyelination in the area of the scar results in denudation of the axonal membrane with resultant pacemaker potentials.[381,382,385] Such irritation of ephaptic burning pain in causalgia is due to nonspecific changes in the environment (temperature change and mechanoreceptor stimulation).

This type of ephaptic pathological pacemaker mechanism is no different than an epileptogenic focus. It causes pathological changes in sodium potassium pump and calcium flux. This principle may explain the beneficial effects of anticonvulsants such as Tegretol® in treatment of ephaptic RSD.[381,385,392–394] The generic form, carbamazepine, is not effective.

A common symptom of ephaptic RSD is aggravation of pain with simple touch with a bed sheet or a mild ambient temperature change or pressure change such as a mild breeze or the weight of a bed sheet. These miniscule stimuli activate the pacemaker potentials.

This focal pacemaker firing explains the reason for the high rate of failure of sympathectomy in treatment of RSD.[341–343,345–360,363,368,370–372]

COMMON AREAS OF EPHAPTIC PAIN

Ephaptic RSD is more commonly seen in *watershed areas*. The watershed areas are the areas of the skin where two or three sensory dermatomal nerves overlap. These are usually over the dorsum of the hand (median, radial, and ulnar nerves) and dorsum of the foot (deep peroneal sural and superficial peroneal nerves).

Usually a small scar in such sensitive areas can cause ephaptic injury and severe RSD.

The destructive nature of the injury also plays a major role in causalgia.

COMMON EPHAPTIC WATERSHED ZONES IN MEDICAL PRACTICE

1. Dorsum of foot: this area is by far the most common site of ephaptic RSD (causalgia). The trauma is usually minor, e.g., an object falling on the foot or a superficial laceration. However, as the scar transgresses the watershed zone (Figures 9a and 9b) of the adjacent sensory nerves (Figure 20), it causes a painful ephapse.

    This condition is aggravated by inappropriate immobilization of the extremity with a cast with resultant additional disuse RSD. Treatment requires a multidisciplinary method. Sympathectomy practically always fails (see Chapter 12).

2. Dorsal and palmar aspect of the hand (Figures 6a and 6b).

3. Ulnar groove at the elbow: blunt or sharp object injury to the ulnar nerve at this area causes ephaptic RSD. This is usually mistaken for tardy ulnar palsy. Surgery is useless for this condition.

4. Sensory nerve injury to the knee due to accidental trauma or arthroscopy being used with increasing frequency is quite difficult to treat.[84]

5. Nerve root contusion (neuropraxia): usually nerve root contusion (Table 7) occurs in the lumbar region even though cervical nerve roots may undergo the same phenomenon. Trauma usually is in the form of a fall on the pelvic region with resultant "guillotine" effect on the nerve root (Tables 9 and 10). MRI or CT are usually negative. Myelography may show "amputation" of the nerve root. At the time of surgery, the nerve root is proximally swollen and distally (at intervertebral foramen level) it is tapered off or

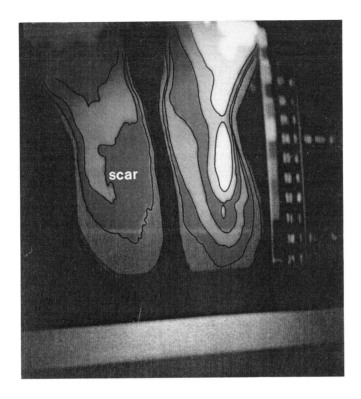

FIGURE 20. Disruption of isothermic lines in ephaptic dystrophy at the watershed zone on dorsum of foot. See also color plates following page 42.

thinned out. Surgery only aggravates the condition by causing inactivity as well as adding the potential for further scar formation. The use of nerve blocks, epidural steroid injections, physiotherapy, ACTH, and antidepressants (e.g., trazodone) provide some relief.

CAUSALGIA

> "A syndrome of sustained burning pain after a traumatic nerve injury combined with vasomotor and sudomotor dysfunction and later trophic changes."
>
> Merskey

Causalgias are divided into two forms:

1. **Causalgia major** involves peripheral nerve injury with electrical "crosstalk" (ephapse) that causes severe hyperactivity of sympathetic system (hyperpathia, vasoconstriction, and movement disorder). The major form is severe, usually caused by injury with high velocity sharp objects (e.g., butcher's knife), vibratory component major trauma (e.g., bullet), or high-voltage nerve lesions (electrocution).
2. **Causalgia minor** involves the same principle as causalgia major, but milder injury, e.g., injury to the dorsum of hand or foot, nerve root contusion, patient falling from a height on gluteal region resulting in "guillotine" effect, bruisng of nerve root caught at the narrowed intervertebral foramen.

The difference between the two categories is a matter of degree and severity.

To classify causalgia as an independent illness is artificial, and **causalgia is nothing but a severe form of RSD**.[340,363–365]

In this severe form of RSD, the course of the disease is quite accelerated from stage 1 through 4 in a matter of weeks or months. S. Weir Mitchell[230] in 1872 first reported rapid development of atrophic changes in the skin, nails, and soft tissues of the extremity in a matter of days to weeks.

Whereas in RSD of disuse the extremity is cold, in ephaptic dystrophy the thermography reveals in the distal portion of the extremely cold extremity that there is an isolated *hot spot* that points to the area of scar formation and ephaptic peripheral nerve dysfunction (Figures 4–6). In this area the vasoconstrictive capability of the sympathetic nerve is paralyzed, and there is a topical hot spot. This hot spot can be appreciated only by thermography.[289]

This type of RSD is quite painful and very difficult to treat. It demands multidisciplinary therapy as well as early diagnosis. The **ephaptic form** is characterized by **increased heat emission** at the area of ephaptic lesion (**electric short**). As the condition becomes chronic, the distal portion of the extremity involved and the contralateral extremity become cold, but the ephaptic spot stays hyperalgesic and warm (Figures 4, 5, 6a, and 6b).

CAUSALGIC PAIN

Sunderland[363] in 1978 succinctly defined causalgic pain as follows:

1. Usually pain occurs after the injury to a nerve trunk.
2. The severity of the injury to the soft tissues other than the nerve does not play a role in the severity of the pain.
3. The pain is spontaneous, severe, and quite persistent.
4. There is a markedly lowered threshold for aggravation of pain. This is the case in all RSD patients, but it is more exaggerated in causalgics. So even a breeze over the skin or the touch of a bed sheet or a change of the environment or a family argument and aggravation can markedly aggravate the pain. This feature of emotional aggravation is

common to all RSD patients, and it is nothing but the role of the frontal lobe and the limbic system in aggravation of hyperpathic pain.

5.   The pain is felt distal to the proximal nerve injury, i.e., in the hand or foot. This is typical but not invariable. The pain does not necessarily have to be a burning type of pain, and can be described in many other hyperpathic forms.

6.   Sunderland established the requirement that the pain should be present for at least 5 weeks. However, depending on the severity of the injury, the pain can develop in a matter of days or weeks. What happens to an extremity in RSD of disuse in a matter of several months can happen in a matter of a few weeks to a causalgic patient.

In no case of RSD is the pain so severe, so intolerable from **burning, seering, aching, tingling, lightening, stabbing, crushing,** to a combination of the above, without burning pain in a matter of a few hours to up to 7 to 10 days in close to 90% of the cases.[374] However, it is not unusual to see some patients who develop the pain as late as 3 to 4 weeks after the injury.[375]

Major causalgia is due to scar formation of peripheral nerves but has a component of **high-velocity or high-vibration injury** in its etiology. This is usually seen after bullet injuries or high-velocity sharp objects such as a butcher knife or surgical instrument injury. This is typically seen in war injuries, but it can also be seen in civilian trauma due to amputation of an extremity or industrial injury to the extremity. It is not uncommon in electrical injuries.

Drilling steel against titanium in the aerospace industry causes high-frequency vibration and makes the patient more susceptible to causalgia.

The difference between the minor and major causalgias is a matter of degree and severity. For more detail on causalgia, see Chapters 1 and 12.

MAJOR CAUSALGIA AND MOTOR DYSFUNCTION

Major causalgia is the best example of efferent dysfunction secondary to sensory nerve damage and RSD. This efferent dysfunction is quite frequently present among causalgic patients (at least over 50% of the patients) and is in the form of flexion deformity of the extremity, tremor, weakness of the extremity, and dystonic movements.

The management of major causalgia requires a multidisciplinary approach. Trigger point injections should be applied to referred pain areas rather than the area of peripheral nerve damage. Repetitive sympathetic nerve blocks can be quite effective. Sympathectomy should be used only for patients who have failed with every other form of therapy and when the patient has a short life expectancy.

Even among patients who have had such a conservative approach toward sympathectomy, there still may be the necessity for morphine pump after failure of sympathectomy (Table 42). Morphine pump, a last resort in treatment, provides good control of pain. As most causalgic patients in civilian (as opposed to war) practice are involved in protracted litigation (especially worker's compensation cases), by the time they are being evaluated for RSD several months or years have elapsed, and the only effective treatment is morphine pump in this stage IV of the disease. For more detail on causalgia, see Chapters 1 and 12.

7

Origins of RSD

PERIPHERAL VS. CENTRAL ORIGIN

Ever since 1872 when S. Weir Mitchell[228,230] first reported RSD, the mechanism of the development of this disease in regard to peripheral or central origin has been the subject of hot debate.

Our present knowledge of the disease shows that the five schools of thought, Mitchell,[228,230] Livingston,[196,197] Ochoa and Torebjork,[251,252] Roberts,[301] and Nathan,[242] which point to the origin of pain anywhere from peripheral nerve to practically all CNS structures, are all valid and describe different aspects of the mechanism of development of RSD (see Chapter 1, History and Figure 1).

MECHANISM OF RSD

PERIPHERAL MECHANISM

The peripheral mechanisms of RSD involve the following:

1. Ephaptic* electrical discharge
2. Ephaptic substance P and norepinephrine secretion
3. "Angry backfiring c fibers"
4. Inactivity due to pain
5. Hypersensitization (Cannon's phenomenon)

The peripheral mechanism is best exemplified in the case of ephaptic RSD. In this condition the secretion of norepinephrine, substance P, and lactic acid, as well as other noxious substances, causes stimulation of the peripheral nerve and input of pain to the central nervous system. If the source of pain becomes chronic and repetitive, then the condition will become self-sustaining (Figures 4–7, 14).

In addition to ephaptic chemical irritation, Ochoa has described the ABC phenomenon (angry backfiring c fibers).[251,252] This abnormal firing of the fibers is one factor in the early development of RSD in ephaptic syndrome. The angry backfiring c fibers result in hyperalgesia and allodynia due to polymodal hyperpathia. This explains why in allodynia even simple touch or slight change of temperature causes severe pain and aggravation of ephaptic RSD.

---

* Ephapse refers to a pathologic electric short in nerve fibers. This is in contrast to synapse, which avoids any electric short by buffer zone of synaptic cleft.

In addition, hypersensitization (Cannon's phenomenon) due to injury to the peripheral nociceptors can cause aggravation of the pain in causalgia and other forms of ephaptic RSD.

Finally, cross-modality threshold modulation (XMT of Ochoa) explains why any change of temperature may aggravate the pain. In such cases with the hyperalgesia, repetitive sympathetic nerve blocks or sympathectomy are apt to fail.

CENTRAL (SPINAL CORD) MECHANISM

The central (spinal cord) mechanisms involve the following:

1. Vicious circle of Livingston
2. Central biasing mechanism of Melzack
3. Turbulance of Sutherland
4. WDR of Nathan

Experimental animal studies have shown CNS changes after peripheral nerve injury.[424–426] Changes have been recorded in spinal cord.[424,425] as well as in cerebral hemispheric cortex.[427] The changes are both electrical as well as chemical, i.e., changes in peptides in cerebral cortex and in spinal cord (CCK, substance P, etc.) especially in the dorsal horn.[426]

The spinal cord plays a major role in modulation of pain and development of RSD. It can be the sole source and point of origination of RSD. This point has been very well demonstrated in spinal cord-injured patients who have no other source of RSD.[71]

Cremer, Maynard, and Davidoff[71] emphasized the development of RSD after spinal cord injury and the need for early diagnosis and early treatment of such patients.

Regardless of peripheral or central points of origination of RSD, the spinal cord exerts a strong modulatory influence on the development and perpetuation of RSD.

The following are some of the mechanisms by which the spinal cord modulates the rate and duration of RSD.

Vicious Circle

Livingston[196,197] was the first to point to hyperactivity of anterolateral horn motor cells in the spinal cord secondary to reduced proprioceptive sensory input (inactivity). The resultant sympathetic hyperactivity causes RSD of disuse (Figures 12a, 12b, and 17).

Microneurographic recordings[396] show a linkage between proprioceptive Pacinian corpuscles and muscle spindle afferent fiber activity and the rate of discharge of efferent sympathetic fibers in humans.[396]

Animal experiments reveal a feedback between cutaneous afferent nerve fibers and sympathetic activity as mentioned above.[396–399]

The vicous circle of Livingston shows the major role of the uninhibited anterolateral horn cells of the spinal cord due to deafferentation and decreased input of proprioception from the extremity to the brain matter of the spinal cord. This decrease of proprioceptive input results in lack of inhibition of the sympathetic nerve cells in the anterolateral horn of spinal cord and hyperactivity of sympathetic nervous system.

Chemical Forms of Vicious Circle

The sympathetic hyperactivity is in three forms:

1. β-Adrenergic, which is a presynaptic phenomenon and is due to stimulation of the preganglionic sympathetic nerve fibers: plays a major role in craniocervical RSD.
2. α-Adrenergic postsynaptic nerve fibers that cause vasoconstriction and muscle spasm.
3. Cholinergic stimulation, which results in hyperhydrosis (excessive sweating), and trophic disturbances of growth of hair and nail.

The best way to manage the vicious circle is physiotherapy, which increases the proprioceptive input and inhibits the hyperactivity of the sympathetic nervous system.

Central Biasing Mechanism

The second mechanism at the spinal cord level is Melzack's gate mechanism and "central biasing mechanism". This phenomenon refers to the fact that the substantia gelatinosa in the posterior horn of the spinal cord acts as a gate inhibiting the input of the pain stimulus into the spinal cord. Stimulation of large fibers inhibits the nociceptive input of c fibers into substantia gelatinosa and blocks the pain and vice versa. This is the principle on which TNS treatment has been developed. Again, TNS and physiotherapy would apply this theory in management of pain and RSD at the spinal cord level.

Turbulence Phenomenon of Sunderland

The third mechanism by which the spinal cord influences pain and RSD is Sunderland's[362,363] turbulence phenomenon. This phenomenon refers to the c fibers stimulating a wide dynamic range (WDR) of neurons in the dorsal horn of the spinal cord with resultant allodynia to the point that even simple touch would cause severe pain in cases of advanced RSD or in cases of early or late ephaptic dystrophy. In this situation, turbulence refers to the fact that ephaptic RSD causes formation of pools of hyperactive dorsal horn cells resulting in perpetuation of turbulence of pain up and down the spinal cord.

WDR

Nathan[242] used the same principle to explain the development of RSD in CNS lesions due to multiple sclerosis or head injuries. Nathan's phenomenon[242] refers to wide dynamic range (WDR) neurons of the dorsal horn cells in the spinal cord or in trigeminal nucleus resulting in the spread and perpetuation of pain without any need for peripheral stimulus to start the pain. The same phenomenon explains the development of craniocervical and craniofacial pain such as seen with head and face injuries resulting in migraine.

Nathan's WDR phenomenon refers to the WDR being at axial as well as vertical levels of substantia gelatinosa. The vertical level extends as far as three adjacent nerve roots in each direction in caudal and cephalad levels. This explains why rhizotomy is useless surgical treatment on a long-term basis.

In multiple sclerosis it is well known that the patient can develop severe trigeminal neuralgia or other types of intractable pain or RSD in the absence of any peripheral nerve injury. Sunderland[363] and Nathan's[242] WDR also explain the reason for the extremely high rate of failure in rhizotomy for treatment of pain.

CENTRAL (BRAIN STEM) MECHANISM

The brain stem originates and perpetuates RSD in head, neck, and face injuries, as well as in the rest of the body.

The role of the **brain stem** in the development and perpetuation of RSD is **multifactorial**. The brain stem is instrumental in **inhibition of pain** input to the higher centers of the brain. It is influential in modulating pain both **electrically** and **chemically**. This modulation is exerted in **ascending (excitatory)** and **descending (inhibitory)** pathways.

Our study of electrical injury patients with RSD shows a high rate of brain stem dysfunction in these patients.[147]

The **chemical influence** is the influence of **substance P, serotonin** (Table 9), as well as **endocrine influence** exerted in the area of the **brain stem**. This endocrine influence is in the form of adjustment of secretion of endorphins as well as ACTH[40] (Figures 21a, 21b, 30, and 31). The central perpetuation of chronic pain and RSD can develop due to inappropriate use of narcotics with resultant reduction of endorphins as well as alcohol and cocaine. Both

TABLE 8
RSD Misdiagnosed as

Migraine	Thoracic outlet syndrome [a]	Shoulder-hand syndrome
Bursitis of shoulder or hip	Myofascial injury	Ligamentous injury
Frozen shoulder	Raynaud's phenomenon	Thalamic pain
Phantom pain	Rotator cuff injury	Aseptic necrosis of hip
Migratory osteolysis	Transient regional osteoporosis	TMJ disease[b]

[a] Nine patients had been previously diagnosed and surgically treated as "thoracic outlet syndrome". The source of pain was cervical nerve root contusion in 4, cervical spondylosis in 2, RSD of disuse in 2, and ephaptic RSD of forearm in 1. Thermography showed RSD changes in all 9 patients. By virtue of muscle spasm involving deltoid, pectoralis, and scalenus muscles, RSD can clinically mimic thoracic outlet syndrome.

[b] RSD causes TMJ disease and vice versa. The two usually coexist. Injections or operation for TMJ disease due to RSD aggravate the condition.

TABLE 9
Low CSF Serotonin

Low CSF serotonin is most frequently associated with
   Violent suicide
   Alcoholism
   Bulimia

From Asberg, et al. (Karolinska Institute) in Meltzer; Psycho-pharmacology. New York: Raven Press, 1987, pp. 655–668.

alcohol and cocaine cause eventual depletion of brain stem catecholamines on a long-term basis.

In addition, the presence of β-adrenergic receptors in the brain stem and the higher centers of the brain shows the importance of the sympathetic nervous system in the control of pain at these levels. The role of RSD in the development of vascular mirgraine headaches will be discussed in the following chapters. This influence is mainly through changes of vascular constriction over the scalp and face due to sympathetic disturbance.

The effect of propranolol on the brain stem also reflects the importance of vascular influence of the brain stem in the modulation of RSD headaches. This is discussed in detail in Chapter 12 on management of RSD.

The Brain Stem as a Modulator of Pain

The brain stem hormonal system, which includes ACTH, endorphin, and leutinizing hormone (LH), is quite instrumental in modulation of pain as described by Melzack and Wall in their wide dynamic range (WDR) theory.

A neurotransmitter, **serotonin** (Table 9), plays a major role in modulation of pain, especially headache. Cholecystokinin (CCK), an octapeptide, is rich in caudal, rhombendephalic heart, and in the bilateral wings of nucleus raphe dorsalis.[276] The rate of concentration of CCK in the brain is influential in threshold of pain perception: the higher the CCK concentration, the higher the pain threshold.*

The Brain Stem as a Modulator of RSD

The brain stem has a dual role in the mechanism of RSD. The first role is the anatomical structure of the reticular system, which has both an excitory and inhibitory effect on the transmission of pain not only through spinoreticular tracts but also through the central biasing feedback mechanism of Melzack.[119]

* CCK concentration in the brain stem and frontal lobe plays a major role in hyperactivity and weight loss. (The higher the CCK concentration, the more active and thinner the animal.)

This central biasing mechanism proposed by Melzack refers to the fact that the large and small fibers activate the neural pools in the spinal cord and brain stem. Each neural pool successively activates and excites the higher levels of neural pools.

The central biasing mechanism of Melzack is influenced both by an inhibitory projection system that originates in the brain stem reticular formation and by excitory spinal reticular fibers that transmit nociceptor pain. This mechanism explains the reason for the failure of sympathectomy in treatment of RSD as well as the persistence of phantom limb pain.

When the sensory nerve fibers of paleonociceptors are destroyed — such as in the case of **sympathectomy** or after **amputation** — there is a **reduction in inhibitory proprioceptive input** on the reticular formation in the brain stem. This results in a **sustained activity** at all levels of the **spinal cord**, **brain stem**, **thalamus**, and **cortex** with aggravation and perpetuation of pain.

The Brain Stem as an Endocrine Center

The second role of the brain stem in modulation of RSD pain is its major role in endocrine influence on pain. The brain stem is quite essential in the formation of endorphins[479] and benzodiazepines (BZ), and the iatrogenic use of exorphins and benzodiazepines (such as diazepam, etc.) causes suppression of formation of endorphins and BZ in the brain stem and results in perpetuation of pain.

The brain stem is practically an extension of the limbic system (Figure 21). It has extensive connections — through neurotransmitters and hormones — with thalamus, hypothalamus, neocortex and paleocortex (limbic system) (Figure 21).

The natural endocrine response of the brain stem to pain is both catabolic and anabolic.

1. Catabolic response is an increase in ACTH, endorphins, cortisone, ADH, growth hormone (GH), cyclic AMP, catecholamines, renin, angiotensin II, interleuken 1, glucagon, and aldosterone.[35]
2. The anabolic endocrine effect of brain stem includes reduction of testosterone, reduction of LH, reduction of estrogens, and decrease in insulin formation. The brain stem plays a role in reduction of insulin through its adrenergic influence on the endocrine system as well as a reduction in male and female hormones through its direct effect on the hypothalamus.[35]

Serotonin and Norepinepherine as Modulators of RSD in Brain Stem

Serotonin is present in the brain stem nuclei. The existence of transmitter-containing cell bodies in the nuclei of the brain of a rat with high serotoninergic innervation has been demonstrated in a large number of brain stem nuclei. Specifically, nucleus raphe magnus and nucleus raphe dorsalis are rich in both serotonin and leuenkephaline.[276]

There are many different forms of serotonin with different physiologic effects.

Serotonins are formed in the brain stem and transmitted to the dorsal roots of the spinal cord. Transmedullary section in rats depletes serotonin in distal levels of dorsal horns.[35]

Vasoactive amines such as serotonin, histamine, catecholamines, and prostaglandins have been blamed for causing and aggravating pain and headache by increasing vasodilation. However, recent studies by Moskowitz,[233–236] Raskin,[287] Olesen,[254] and Aghajanian and Wang[5] emphasize the importance of serotonin as a neurotransmitter in raphe nuclei of the brain stem as the modulator of pain such as migraine headaches.

Serotonin has contrasting effects at presynaptic and postsynaptic levels. As early as 1961, Sicuteri[337] reported a rise in the 5-hydroxy indoleacetic acid (5-HIAA) which is a byproduct of serotonin in the urine of migraine patients during headache attacks. More recent studies by Anthony[11] demonstrated that during migraine attacks the platelet serotonin levels fall simul-

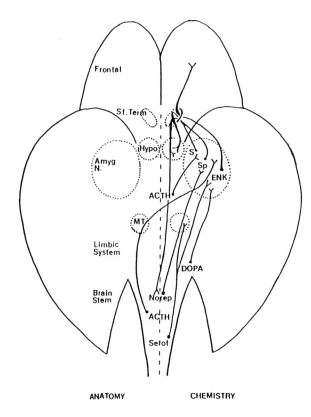

ANATOMY   CHEMISTRY

FIGURE 21a. Brain stem as an extension of the limbic system and endocrine system. Some of the chemicals generated and distributed from brain stem to the rest of the limbic system and to the thalamic and hypothalamic nuclei.[92]

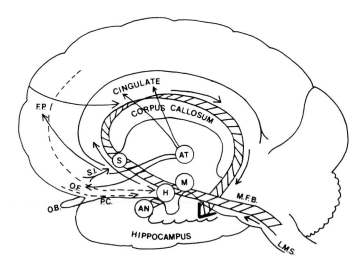

FIGURE 21b. A major portion of the limbic system is located in the brain stem. Through the median forebrain bundle (M.F.B.) this portion of the brain stem interacts with the rest of the limbic system as far up as the frontal polar region, orbital frontal region, cingulate gyrus, and hippocampus. This system intermingles emotions, moods, memory, and the autonomic responses as the interaction of the conscious reflexive cerebral functions. (Modified from Kelly.[439])

taneously with an increase in serotonin levels in the urine. The highest concentration of serotonin (over 90%) is in the wall of the intestine. Less than 10% of serotonin in the body is present in the brain and is mainly in the raphe nuclei of the brain stem as well in gray matter of spinal cord.

Methysergide acts as a serotonin antagonist in CNS and relieves vascular headaches between attacks. In contrast to sumptriptan and ergotamines, it has no effect on an acute ongoing attack. It has an inhibitory influence on brain stem nuclei. This inhibitory effect is mainly on the presynaptic function of serotonin. Periactin and methysergide, the antagonists of presynaptic serotonin, reduce the excitability of the raphe nuclei of the brain stem. Electrical stimulation of the raphe nuclei stimulates the formation of serotonin and the release of serotonin to the extracellular synaptic cleft.

An increased concentration of serotonin in the synaptic cleft results in a decrease of presynaptic activity of the serotoninergic neurons in the raphe nuclei. The same phenomenon can be achieved by the use of some antidepressents that reduce the reuptake of serotonin from the synaptic cleft or by monoaminoxidase inhibitors (e.g., phenelzine) that block the breakdown of synaptic cleft serotonin with a secondary suppression of the electrical firing rate of raphe nuclei.

Caffeine and papaverine inhibit the breakdown of cyclic amp postsynaptically and slow down the effect of serotonin at the postsynaptic level with a secondary increase of serotonin at the synaptic cleft.

It becomes obvious that a reduction in synaptic cleft serotonin levels by any cause (trauma, heredity, or toxic agents, such as alcohol and reserpine) results in a higher rate of firing by the raphe nuclei and a lower threshold for pain, especially migraine vascular headaches.[233–236,286–288]

Dietary factors such as administration of tyramine-stimulating foods (red meat and sharp cheese), stimulants such as chocolate (phenethylamine), nitrites, and MSG have similar effects of depletion of synaptic cleft serotonin with resultant aggravation of vascular headaches.

The β blockers such as propranolol and calcium channel blockers (diltiazem hydrochloride, nifedipine, verapamil) seem to slow down the synaptic cleft turnover, and in this regard are beneficial in treatment of migraine headaches and other forms of painful RSD. Dietary components rich in tryptophan, such as mild cheese, yogurt, and buttermilk, are used by presynaptic nerve endings as precursors of serotonin. They result in an increased synaptic cleft serotonin formation, and, as a result, reduce the firing of raphe nuclei.

This seems to be the reason for the antidepressant as well as sedative effect of L-tryptophan and its effect in raising the threshold of pain, be it in the form of migraine or other types of chronic pain (RSD, etc.).

Serotonin in CNS has the opposite effect on pain as serotonin in extracellular spaces in the rest of the body (90% of body serotonin is concentrated in the gastrointestinal system). The release of serotonin into the circulation sensitizes the vessel walls and produces a sterile inflammatory action that causes severe migraine headaches.[283] The same phenomenon occurs in RSD in other parts of the body.

There are other chemicals that play major roles — such as prostaglandins, substance P, and rogue oxygen — in pain of RSD and sterile inflammation of the extravascular areas. Substance P is a ubiquitous substance that is present in CNS as well as other parts of the body. Application of this substance to the eye results in conjunctivitis, vasodilation, myosis, leakage of protein from plasma, and disturbance of the blood-aqueous barrier.[282,283] In contrast to serotonin, dorsal horn nerve cells locally form and transmit substance P (sP) down the nerve roots. Serotonin, on the other hand, is formed in brain stem and transmitted to the dorsal horn of the spinal cord.

This inflammatory substance (sP) not only plays a role in modulation of pain in CNS, but also plays a role in the development of trigger points. Gentle pressure on the trigger point releases substance P, lactic acid, and other irritants that are encapsulated in the trigger point. As a result, the area of the trigger point becomes reddish after gentle pressure. Similar pressure on the corresponding structures across the midline does not cause a reddish (sterile) inflammation. This maneuver helps identify the trigger point. It also explains why even sticking a needle in the trigger point without injection of any substance relieves the pain. This kind of injection releases the encapsulated pain chemicals and makes them accessible for absorption by blood circulation.

Medications Affecting Serotonin in Trigeminovascular RSD (Migraine Headaches)

Drugs that release serotonin precipitate migraine attacks.[183,184] The central serotoninergic nerves (especially originating from the raphe median) influence intracranial vascular caliber as well as transmission of pain in brain and peripheral nerves.[546,547]

Serotonin receptors	Drugs affecting receptors
Serotonin I-D:[548] presynaptic	Ergots, sumatriptan
Serotonin 2:[549] postsynaptic (influence prevention)	Methysergide, cycloheptadine, pizotyline

Brain Stem and Trigeminal Nerve

Besides the above putative influences that the brain stem exerts on RSD type of pain, one other anatomical structure (trigeminal nerves — nuclei) complicates the subject of pain and RSD in its relationship to facial and craniocervical pain.

Superimposed on the complex structure of the brain stem is the vast anatomical structure of the trigeminal nervous system. This system is rich in both somesthetic and sympathetic nerves. Injuries to the face, neck, and scalp result in stimulation of both systems in the trigeminal nerve distribution. This in turn arouses the brain stem in a stronger fashion than similar injuries to the upper and lower extremities (Figures 15 and 21).

The sympathetic system in the distribution of trigeminal nerves follow the same path as the paleospinothalamic tract (PSTT) and directly stimulates the limbic system as well as the cerebral cortex (Figure 15). This stimulation is both ipsilateral and contralateral in contrast to somesthetic fibers, which discretely stimulate the contralateral sensory cortex (Figures 12 and 15).

This stimulation of the limbic system explains the hyperpathia and allodynia that are accompanied by posttraumatic headaches, i.e., vascular migraine type of headaches after head, neck, or face injuries.

RSD AND MIGRAINE

The literature is replete with scattered information regarding causes and mechanisms of development of migraine. Unfortunately the mechanism of development has been mistaken for the cause of migraine, and the mechanism of development has become the center of attention at the expense of ignoring the etiologies of migraine.

Physicians have been enthralled with different manifestations of migraine and have superficially classified different types of migraine headaches according to the severity of clinical manifestations.

However, this does not deny the fact that classifying different degrees of migraine into common, classical, etc., is no different than classifying different manifestations of epilepsy into grand mal, petit mal, etc. Both of them are artificial, superficial, and ignore the original cause.

BRAIN STEM AND MIGRAINE: TRIGEMINOVASCULAR REFLEX

Migraine study has taken a back seat to other types of pain. Both in curriculum of medical schools and in research laboratories there has been a policy of benign neglect toward the study of headaches.

Headaches have been artificially classified as *muscle tension headaches* and *migraine headaches*.

Commonly, the vascular headaches cause more muscle contraction than the muscle-tension headaches. Our EMG studies show more severe and more pathological muscle contraction (usually unilateral cervical paraspinal spasm) in vascular headaches than in tension headaches (with EMG manifestation of mild bilateral cervical paraspinal spasm). So the generally accepted classification of headaches is artificial and nonscientific. There is no doubt that migraine headache is an all or none phenomenon and has nothing in common with muscle tension headache. However, both kinds of headache are nothing but an effect and cannot be considered causative to name a disease after them.

Biofeedback for relief of muscle contraction helps migraine patients more than tension headache patients.

The common denominator in chronic headache patients is a high rate of depression and prevention of headaches with antidepressant therapy.

In posttraumatic migraine headache due to injury to head, face, or neck, stimulation of the sympathetic nervous system to the nociceptors of the trigeminal nerves plays a major role in the development of headache.

The review of experimental studies in migraine research[233,236,422] has demonstrated that certain monoaminergic brain stem nuclei can influence cerebral circulation. Such nuclei through excitation of the trigeminal nerve control and influence the diameter of the external carotid artery. This trigeminovascular reflex plays a major role in the development of migraine headaches. Descending pathways from the same brain stem nuclei induce the adrenal gland to secrete norepinephrine and in turn causes release of serotonin from platelets in the blood.

The platelet serotonin depletion has been demonstrated to instigate vascular headaches in a normal individual as well as migrainous patients. These research works that implicate the brain stem directly in the development of migraine headache show quite important and promising potential for management of migraine headache.

The serotonin agonists such as sumatriptan, a 5-HT1 agonist,[360,361] and imigran are useful in management of migraine and cluster headaches. Intravenous treatment with sumatriptan can significantly relieve attacks of migraine.[361] The 5-HT2 agonists such as pizotifen help prevent migraine attacks.

TRIGEMINOVASCULAR SYSTEM AND MIGRAINE

Extensive studies by Moskowitz[233–236] and earlier works by Ray and Wolff[292] removed any doubt regarding the important role of trigeminal vascular anatomical structures and pathways in the development of migraine headaches.

Moskowitz has done extensive work in pathogenesis of migraine.[53,195,233–236,313] According to his research, the major factor in the development of migraine headache is not simple vasoconstriction and vasodilatation but the **influence of the trigeminal nerve** on the **release of neurotransmitters** and chemicals such as **substance P** and **neurokinin**.

Moskowitz emphasized the role of neurogenically induced substances in the trigeminal ganglion in the development of migraine headaches. The trigeminal nerve plays a major role in control of the blood system diameters in the cranial blood vessels.[422] It also is the afferent pathway for the transmission of head pain.

This role is through transmission from the sympathetic afferent fibers from the sheath of the craniocervical blood vessels to the brain.[422] These fibers stimulate a complex response in the brain stem and cerebral cortex.

Substance P, neurokinin A, and **calcitonin-generated peptides** (CGRP)[53,195,313] are some of the neurotransmitters that are released after **stimulation of the trigeminal vascular system**, and result in a neurogenic type of inflammation in the soft tissues around the wall of the blood vessels with resultant vicious circle of self-perpetuating pain. Not only do these neurotransmitters result in vasodilation but they also cause a leakage of proteins from blood vessels with secondary activation of mass cells.

One byproduct of these processes is the formation of the **superoxide anion radical**. The production of this radical results in release of hydrogen peroxide by dismutation, which secondarily causes vascular and soft tissue injuries and aggravation of severe craniofacial pain, which is clinically diagnosed as migraine. Dr. Moskowitz suggested a neuropathophysiological model for the development of headache pain and the action of antiheadache drugs.

The best way to explain this mechanism — so brilliantly described by Dr. Moskowitz — is the role of trigeminal transmitted reflex sympathetic dysfunction. This explains the classic hyperpathia and hyperalgesia typical of migraine.

The spontaneous improvement of migraine with aging is understood by the fact that the nerve endings of the sympathetic nerve fibers become atrophic. Cranial blood vessels become less sensitive to vasodilation, and as Schmidt et al.[325] have demonstrated, the nerve cell terminals in sympathetic ganglia become extensively swollen and degenerated, responding poorly to sympathetically mediated pain (SMP).

MIGRAINE AND ISCHEMIA

In regard to the mechanism of the development of migraine, there are two major schools of thought. First is the ischemic school, blaming migraine on vasospasm, and second is the CNS school, which tries to find the cause and mechanism of the development of migraine in the central nervous system.

By following reflex sympathetic dystrophy as a model for the mechanism of development of migraine, everything falls in place, and it becomes obvious that vasospasm in the central as well as peripheral nervous systems is an integral part of migraine development.

Like any other type of hyperpathic pain originating from the sympathetic nervous system, the patient's personality, family tendency for low threshold for pain, and peripheral nerve injury in the form of injuries to cervicotrigeminal distribution all play major roles in the development of migraine. In this regard, migraine becomes a multifactorial syndrome that covers the entire spectrum of the clinical manifestations of RSD.

This study of migraine through the RSD theory is not an academic exercise. It helps us approach migraine management in a more comprehensive fashion. Just as RSD should not be a justification for amputation of the extremity, any form of surgical procedure obviously becomes useless for treatment of migraine.

The same medications that temporarily help migraine but aggravate it in the long term (narcotics, barbiturates, benzodiazepines) are also contraindicated in any form of chronic pain including the emotionally laden RSD.

The ischemic school of mechanism of migraine has been best presented by Olesen.[252–254] In his studies he noticed the slowly spreading oligemia involving the cerebral cortex starting at the occipital pole and gradually moving forward. This slowly progressive oligemia, obviously a function influenced by CNS, is very similar to spreading depression of Leao.[553]

Olesen[255–257] and Welch[402] emphasized the **importance of stress** as a precipitating factor in the development of **migraine**.

In Welch's theoretical model[402] the major pathways are identical to the PSTT (Figure 14). "Activity in this pathway triggers activity in intrinsic noradrenergic system."[402]

The activator for development of migraine according to the above authors may be visual through the spreading depression starting from the cerebral cortex or may be somesthetic, such as injuries of the head, face, or cervical spine.

The **spreading depression**[553] provides the missing link in the chain of events of development of **migraine** headache after the origination of vasoconstrictive stimulation in the trigeminal nerve distribution. This vasoconstrictive phenomenon is typical of RSD in any other part of the body, which results in release of substance P and norepinephrine to initiate vasoconstriction as well as vascular permeability, prostaglandin synthesis in the periarterial space, and the development and spread of pain.

SUBSTANCE P

Substance P (sP), a small polypeptide, has been demonstrated to be present in a diffuse fashion in the CNS and peripheral nervous system. It is mostly accumulated and formed in the posterior horn of the gray matter of the spinal cord. The substance P-containing nerve fibers are quite prevalant in the paravertebral sympathetic ganglia of the rat, cat, and guinea pig.[233]

Substance P, an undecapeptide, is seen in abundant concentration in the dorsal horn of the spinal cord as well as in the spinal ganglia of the SNS and in the trigeminal nucleus.[139–141,195,204,271]

Substance P and norepinephrine are the two excitatory substances for the transmission of pain.

In the ascending excitatory and descending inhibitory pathways that modulate the pain, there is a fine balance between the polypeptide (sP) and monoamine norepinephrine on the one side and the inhibitory descending polypeptides, endorphins, and monoamine serotonin on the other.

Whereas the latter inhibitory substances are formed in the higher centers of the brain and are transmitted to the dorsal horn of the spinal cord, the excitatory sP is formed in abundance in the gray matter of the spinal cord and transmitted to the higher centers as well as the spinal ganglia of the SNS and the peripheral nervous system (PNS).[139–141]

The substance P in these ganglia is mainly accumulated in thin and varicose structures representing nerve terminals.

These fibers are also present in the perivascular structures of trigeminal vascular arteriolar branches. It has been suggested that the peripheral branches of substance P-containing primary sensory neurons[234,235] terminate in the paravertebral sympathetic ganglia as well as run through them on their way to the central nervous system. Retrograde tracing experiments with horseradish peroxidase have provided direct evidence for a connection between dorsal root ganglia and paravertebral sympathetic ganglia.[90]

The spreading depression and oligemia can be severe enough to cause hypoxia and migraine headache with resultant hyperaggregation of platelets. This can become severe enough to result in neurologic deficit such as ischemic partial stroke or seizure disorder, which can complicate migraine.[236,403]

Substance P and Sympathetic Ganglia

The sympathetic ganglia are rich in peptides: sP, enkephalin, somatostatin, and vasoactive intestinal peptides (VIP).

Of the monoamine group of transmitters, norepinephrine and serotonin are present in the same ganglia. The largest concentration of serotonin is in the enteric wall and in the enteric nervous system. However, serotonin has multiple contrasting functions in the PNS as contrasted with the CNS. Even in the CNS, serotonin has different functions in different structures and in different illnesses. In CNS, PNS, and SNS, γ-aminobutyric acid (GABA) is present as another inhibitory substance.

Substance P and Headache

The neural connections between trigeminal ganglia and cerebral blood vessels (trigeminal vascular system) constitute the main role in the development of vascular headaches. Moskowitz[236] demonstrated that when the trigeminal vascular system is depolarized, sP is transmitted from trigeminal neurons into the wall of the cerebral blood vessels.

Joseph et al.[472] have shown an increased number of nerve fibers around the blood vessels containing a rich supply of sP in the skin biopsy of cluster headache patients as compared to the normal control group.

Substance P and CNS

The main source of sP is the spinal cord; however, it has been found in the brain in the areas of the basal ganglia, hypothalamus, and substantia nigra.

Substance P increases plasma prolactin. The significance of this elevation of this hormone is not known.

The presence of sP in the nucleus tractus solitarius may point to its influence on baroreceptor reflexes. In Shy-Drager syndrome, the sP level of CSF is reduced. This may be a reflection of a lower level of sP in the peripheral nerves and sympathetic ganglia[473] (see also RSD and migraine sections).

Substance P can be measured in the CSF. It is not only elevated in the CSF of chronic pain patients, but also in patients suffering from other neurologic diseases such as multiple schlerosis.[492]

ROLE OF FRONTAL LOBE IN RSD AND MIGRAINE

In this book we have avoided the use of the term "autonomic nervous system". It is true that the autonomic nervous system exerts a great degree of autonomy regarding blood pressure, pulse, and respiration control. However, this system is not truly independent and autonomous.

The sympathetic system is controlled and influenced at all levels of the central nervous system. It is a feedback system that intermingles the cerebral function from the most primitive to the most complex conscious aspects. If there is any example to refute the concept of psyche vs. soma, sole vs. brain, and organic vs. "psychic" or "functional", it is the way the SNS works.

Experiments on animals reveal that the control of sympathetic system is not achieved by independent "centers" in the spinal cord, medulla, midbrain, thalamus, or cortex. Instead, the entire CNS axis functions as a coordinating unit (Appenzeller[441]). In hypoxic cardiovascular stress, the cortical and the suprapontine centers are activated for proper response (Korner and

Uther[442]). Conversely, the frontal lobe has rich projections directly to the hypothalamic and limbic systems all the way down to the limbic midbrain region.

In this fashion, the frontal polar and frontal orbital regions become contiguous with the limbic system (Nauta[440]) as shown in Figures 21a and 21b adapted from Kelly.[439]

"A defense reaction" circuit from the hypothalamus through the stria terminalis to the amygdaloid nucleus and back is responsible for alertness and defensive attack by the animal. Simultaneously the sympathetic system is stimulated with changes in heart, respiration, and blood pressure for "fight or flight" response. This response is determined by the interaction of the frontal and temporal lobes.[443]

Hughlings Jackson (1931)[444] noted blood pressure and vascular changes due to the pathology of the cerebral cortex in **epileptic** and **brain tumor patients**. Frontal cortical as well as anterior temporal lesions in **frontal lobotomy** and **temporal lobotomy** patients cause blood pressure and pulse changes as well.[445,446] Stimulation of the **cingulate gyrus** results in affective changes as well as blood pressure and pulse changes.[455]

Moreover, the circuit shown in Figures 21a and 21b connecting **hippocampus, temporal lobe**, and **mammilar bodies (Papez circuit)** influences the sympathetic function and provides the emotional basis for retention of immediate recall and short memory. Any **lesion** in this circuit **disturbs the memory function**.[439] **Serotonin** plays a major role in the sympathetic function of the frontal-temporal lobes: activation of cerebral cortical serotonin receptors may raise or reduce systemic blood pressure. **As the serotonin concentration of cerebral cortex increases, the sympathetic function decreases**. This has a protective effect in animals against the development of ventricular fibrillation.[447] This may somehow be useful in **prevention of fatal heart attack**.

As is the case with other forms of RSD, migraine has multiple sites of origin. Another main feature that seems to be the common causative factor in both migraine as well as in other manifestations of RSD is the role of the frontal cortex in response to distress. It is well known that stress is the major aggravating, if not at times the causative factor, for both migraine headache and RSD.

The pioneer work by Skinner and Welch[345] reveals that the neurons in the frontal cortex undergo an event-related slow potential shift (ERSP) in response to a tone that gives the forewarning of cutaneous shock.[343,344] An increase in neural activity and neural firing of the frontal lobe is also reported in the same experiments.[343–346]

In our studies of patients suffering from electrical injuries,[147] RSD is frequently present in the areas of electrical damage (see Etiology of RSD). In some of these patients, the pain becomes quite intractable, and RSD becomes extremely difficult to control. Such patients on topographic brain mapping[149,151] show frontal lobe dysfunction in the form of α dislocation in the frontal lobe area (Figure 23).

Skinner et al.[343,345] and Welch[402,403] consider the frontal lobe as the site of cerebral dysfunction in experiments on cutaneous shocks on animals as well as in migraine. Meyer et al.[225] in their PET studies of cerebral blood flow after vibrotactile stimulation to the fingers of the hand not only recorded contralateral somatosensory (parietal) cortex selective increase of cerebral blood flow but demonstrated an ipsilateral frontal polar cortex increase of cerebral blood flow reflecting modulation of the human cortex response by the attentive behavior of the subject with respect to the stimulus.

The above-mentioned studies have in common activation of the part of the frontal lobe that is usually activated by PSTT fibers, especially in a pathologic fashion in RSD patients. Both migraine and RSD patients have an alarmist and hyperpathic response to their pain.

This alarm response has the common sites of anterior and mesial frontal regions (Figures 14 and 23). This area of the brain is mainly activated by the cortical noradrenergic neurotransmitter system. In migraine the noradrenergic β-receptor function is quite essential for visual cortex neurons to be physiologically programmed by a change in visual input.

Following the model proposed by Welch[402,403] and considering the spreading depression as well as the oligemic response in migraine demonstrated by Olesen,[255] a link is noted between the orbital-frontal lobes and the alarm response of sympathetic vascular pain and headache. The noradrenergic β-receptor function is necessary for certain visual cortex neurons to be physiologically programmed by a change in visual input.

Injection of β-blockers into the orbital-frontal brain stem projection areas alters the autonomic out-flow both in regard to its initiation in the frontal lobes and its relay into the brain stem.[346]

LIMBIC SYSTEM, RSD, AND MIGRAINE

The rich connections of the paleospinothalamic tract originating in the trigeminal nuclei with the limbic system (temporal lobe, frontal lobe, and brain stem) result in a diffused type of vascular headache. This type of hyperpathia at times has a hereditary pattern, and in at least one out of four migraine headache patients, there is definitely a strong family history of migraines. However, this does not mean that every member of the family is going to develop migraines. Frequently a minor injury to the head, face, or neck in a patient who has this type of diasthesis results in the development of migraine in family members.

Using the above experimental models that have been developed by Welch and Skinner, it becomes quite clear that we are not dealing with coincidence of migraine and RSD functioning through identical areas of the brain and causing identical similar pictures with different terminology.

PERIPHERAL CERVICOFACIAL (REFERRED PAIN) MIGRAINE

The third mechanism of involvement of trigeminal nerve and RSD in the development of migraine headaches is on the principle of referred pain. As demonstrated by Ruch,[310] the referred pain from areas adjacent to the head and face initiate from referred pain over the head and face, which is accompanied by RSD changes typical of migraine headache. Ruch's theory is nothing more than the famous physiologist, Sherrington's neural pool concept. Sherrington's[573] principle is based on the fact that several c fibers converge on the few nerve cells in the dorsal horn through the posterior roots (Figure 15). This convergence of the few nerve cells that originate in the spinothalamic tract results in convergence on several nerve fibers from different adjacent areas on the same set of neurons. As a result, there are superimposed neural pools as specified by Sherrington in the form of A, B, and C cycles superimposing each other, which would comprise the spinothalamic tract neurons in a segment of the spinal cord (Figure 15).

For example, an injury to the upper cervical spine at the level of the C2 or C3 posterior arch of the spine or articular facets results in convergence of the sensory nerve fibers from these areas on the substantia gelatinosa of C1 and C2 levels of the spinal cord. The same substantia gelatinosa is the nucleus for the spinothalamic tract of the trigeminal nerve. As a result, the upper cervical spine injuries result in severe referred pain over the area of the ophthalmic branch of the trigeminal nerve with typical visual aura of migraine vascular headache and typical throbbing pain over the retroorbital frontal region of the head (Figure 16).

The best clues for cervicogenic migraine are as follows (Table 10):

1. Aggravation or initiation of migraine with weather change (drop in barometric pressure causes vacuum effect in C spine joints and initiates the referred pain of migraine).
2. Careful cervical spine examination and search and injection of trigger points over the articular facets results in successful treatment of cervicogenic migraine.
3. Application of craniocervical thermography identifies cervical spine soft tissue pathology in over one third of all migraine patients.
4. The application of antiinflammatory medications such as naproxine or injection of stadol results in excellent control of cervicogenic migraine patients.

The fact that many such patients also have migrainous diathesis and a strong family history of migraine results in a cursory examination by the clinician and treatment of headache as migraine headache with dangerous medications such as methysergide or propranolol. In such cases, at times, a simple trigger point injection over the cervical paraspinal articular facets can

TABLE 10
Symptoms of Cervicogenic Migraine[a]

Migraine starts or gets worse with drop in barometric pressure[b]
Migraine starts or is worse toward the end of a long working day
Shooting pain in retroorbital and occipital regions (referred pain from cervical spine)
Migraine in a patient with a long history of surgical procedures for thoracic outlet syndrome, carpal tunnel
    syndrome, tardy ulnar palsy, rotator cuff tear, etc.
Resurgence of migraine after several years of remission after age 45 and after menopause
Patient pointing to suboccipital region as the point of origination of headache. Usually this area has a trigger
    point due to old trauma. Injection of the trigger point over C2, C3, or C4 neural arch produces excellent
    relief

[a] The above symptoms should point to cervical spondylosis or old cervical sprain. Posterior cervical trigger points
     are quite common among these patients. Cervical traction and trigger point injection result in excellent relief of
     headache.
[b] As is the case with all other joint diseases, a drop in barometric pressure causes a vacuum effect in the synovia
     of joints, and edema ex vacuo causes pain in cervical spine joints.

get rid of the pain much easier than trying to treat patients as if they had idiopathic migraine headaches.

Of 100 patients diagnosed with migraine headache, only 25% fall into the classic category of migraine headaches. The other 75% frequently have other sources of pain such as cervical spine injury, injury to the soft tissues of the neck, scars over the scalp, and other injuries resulting in RSD in the head and face regions.

One of the earliest uses of thermography was in the study of sympathetic changes accompanying migraine headache as early as the 1960s. Thermography can be quite useful in detecting the origin of RSD, which can mimic migraine headache secondary to head, face, or posterior cervical injuries. Thermography should be done of the head and face and posterior cervical regions (Figures 2a, 18a, and 18b).

Recognizing the above mechanism of cervical spine origin of vascular headaches is rewarded by successful management of migraine with physiotherapy, cervical traction, and articular facet trigger point injections.

The use of cervicofacial thermography can shed light on the nature of migraine in such patients (Figures 27–29).

8

Referred Pain and Trigger Point

REFERRED PAIN

Referred pain usually accompanies RSD. The acute non-RSD (somesthetic) type of pain usually is not accompanied by referred pain.

Referred pain is quite common in visceral pathology. Whereas burning, crushing, and cutting of skin cause severe pain, the same stimuli do not cause any sensation in the gut.[432] The noxious stimuli that cause pain and referred pain in the viscera are distention,[431] anoxia,[436] and acidity.[434]

Lewis[433] demonstrated that stimulation of "myofascial" structures, i.e., muscle, periosteum, and ligaments, causes pain quite similar to visceral pain. Lewis[433] stimulated referred pain in 94% of experimental injections of 6% normal saline into deep skeletal structures of 28 normal volunteers. The pattern of referred pain was quite consistent, although not confined to the injected dermatomal segment. Cohen,[429] Theobald,[437] and White and Sweet[438] demonstrated that superficial stimulation of peripheral lesions (e.g., a fractured elbow or a stump neuroma) can instigate recurrence of angina pectoris. It is obvious that cutaneous stimulation causes efferent visceral changes such as vasoconstriction. This referred pain, typical of the function of the sympathetic system, is quite common in RSD (e.g., shoulder-hand syndrome). It may explain the higher incidence of heart attack in RSD patients. Obviously stress-induced pain (SIP) is another feature of RSD that results in distressful strain on the cardiovascular system.

Sterling phenomenon[435] has been experienced by the majority of the normal population. This referred pain is a sharp pain — always ipsilateral and in a distant dermatome — after scraping of the skull with a fingernail or pulling of an unwanted hair (e.g., nostril hair). The same phenomenon is noted pathologically on dilatation of abdominal aneurysm, which can cause pain in the testicle prior to sudden death. Squeezing the testicle can cause an excruciating pain in the nipple.

Most commonly, referred pain occurs in cervical spondylosis (see Etiology of RSD) and cervial sprain with complex symptoms outlined in the section on cervical spondylosis in Table 13.

The two factors that are important in the development of referred pain are (1) **wide dynamic range** (WDR) **distribution** of c fibers at the point of input in the spinal cord and (2) **Sherrington's phenomenon**[573] (Figure 16).

As the physiologist Sherrington demonstrated,[573] referred pain is principally caused by the input of multiple sensory nerves from different dermatomes and different parts of the body

83

(skin as well as viscera) into substantia gelatinosa in the dorsal horn of the spinal cord (Figures 10, 11, 13, and 16).

The large number of sensory nerve endings entering the substantia gelatinosa stimulate fewer number of internuncial nerve cells. This results in an overlap of sensory input — be it proprioceptive or nociceptive — on the same secondary neurons (Figure 16).

The overlap results in the stimulation of one nerve cell by multiple nerves. For example, a nociceptive input from an inflamed appendix may overlap the proprioceptive input of proximal portions of the ileum. As a result, the appendicitis pain may be felt in the epigastric region.

These dorsal branches of the posterior cervical nerve roots overlap the distal branches of the same nerve roots at the area of entrance to the substantia nigra. As a result, a patient who has nerve root irritation may not feel the pain in the hand or arm, but in the posterior aspect of the shoulder (Figure 16). This results in mistaken diagnoses such as bursitis of the shoulder or rotator cuff injury.

The same principle of referred pain can result in an increase or decrease in temperature in the trigger points in the remote areas of sensory nerve endings. For example, damage over the dorsum of the hand to the radial nerve may cause increased temperature in the distribution of sensory nerve fibers of the radial nerve in the dorsum of the hand, and may also cause a trigger point of hot or cold nature in the posterior aspect of the shoulder.

Usually the trigger point is cold (Figures 2a and 3). It is commonly seen in the posterior aspect of the shoulder, trapezius muscle, scalene muscle, sacroiliac joint region, or frontal region of the head in the case of upper cervical nerve irritation (Figure 5) where they are cold rather than hot spots. The cold trigger point is formed by longstanding myofascial reaction to the accumulation of substance P and other irritants in the area of referred pain.

Massage or insertion of a needle in the cold spot results in release of the entrapped irritants. The superimposed skin becomes reddish, and after several minutes the irritants are absorbed. This may be the reason for therapeutic effects of massage.

TRIGGER POINT AND MYOFASCIAL PAIN

Myofascial pain refers to a source of pain originating from muscle under fascia in any part of the body.

Unfortunately, this terminology has been abused so extensively that it has lost its meaning. It is mainly being used by unsophisticated clinicians to refer to any kind of pain that they cannot understand.

The true myofascial pain, which refers to origination of pain in the muscle under the fascia, is a typical trigger point (TP).

Due to abuse of terminology, we shall avoid any reference to myofascial type of pain. The following discussion addresses only the subject of trigger point.

Trigger point (Figures 2a, 3, 22) is a painful spot that is usually cold. Pressure on the trigger point results in a reddish discoloration and temporary aggravation of pain followed by relief after injection or massage of the point. Trigger point has been recognized as a phenomenon for several decades. It has been utilized in management of the patient in disciplines such as medicine, osteopathy, and chiropractic. Its scientific recognition and classification as well as an explanation of the phenomenon were first described in a classic academic style by Travell in 1976.[376,377] Prior to her classification, other terminologies were used and reported as early as 1900.[116,123,156,324,376,377]

Trigger point is an area of pain in the muscle that is usually some distance away from the original pathologic condition originating the pain. Trigger point is quite a common phenomenon. Only recently has any significant attention been paid to trigger point.

MECHANISM OF FORMATION OF TRIGGER POINT

The trigger point has numerous causes. Anything that causes referred pain can manifest itself in the form of trigger point.

The trigger point can be cold, which is usually the case (lower temperature than the surrounding tissues). On occasion it may be hot, showing an increased temperature in the area of TP (Figures 2a, 2b, 3).

The TP is usually cold because of the fact that the TP is accompanied by vasospasm in the muscle. The same vasospasm decreases the temperature and causes hypoxia and pain in the area. The TP usually accumulates painful substances (substance P, lactic acid, etc.). The surrounding vasoconstriction causes entrapment of the painful substances.

Certain areas of the body are more prone to developing trigger points. It is most commonly seen over the **articular facet joints of spine.**

Trigger point is quite commonly a complication of RSD. Thermography usually shows a cold spot in the area of the TP, but a hot spot can occasionally be seen due to the fact that the severity of the pathology has resulted in a vasodilation following longstanding vasoconstriction (Figure 7).

Bedside examination of the trigger point shows moderate pain and tenderness. Rubbing the trigger point with the examiner's fingers almost invariably changes a cold spot to a hot spot. This helps identify the location of the TP for injection. Except for thermography, which at times identifies the TP, no other laboratory test can help identify this phenomenon (Figures 2a, 2b, 3).

The patient's symptomatology and a careful neurologic examination are the best tools in the diagnosis of TP short of thermography.

As is the case with RSD, TP pain also is misdiagnosed with synonyms such as bursitis, shoulder-hand syndrome, atypical facial pain, tendonitis, occipital neuralgia, rotator cuff syndrome, thoracic outlet syndrome, myofascial pain, arthritis, tennis elbow, epicondylitis, ligamentous injury, migraine headache, and a variety of other names.

Some of the names mentioned above, such as rotator cuff tear and cervical sprain, may be the cause of trigger point. But other names are used because of the fact that the clinician does not recognize the TP.

CLINICAL DIAGNOSIS OF TRIGGER POINT

The TP may be active or latent. The active TP is a hyperactive focus of pain in the muscle usually accompanied by other forms of autonomic disorder (RSD) and is easy to diagnose.

The latent TP is diagnosed only during the examination. Even though it causes delayed pain in the surrounding area, the latent TP is best diagnosed by careful palpation of the soft tissues. This is especially the case in the shoulder and neck areas.

A careful cervical paraspinal muscle area examination is essential in the diagnosis of not only ligamentous injuries but also in identification of TP. This should be done on every migraine patient.

When the TP is identified, proper treatment of the TP can result in a practically complete cessation of headache, neck pain, or shoulder pain.

Palpation of the TP area and pressure on the spot reproduces pain as well as the referred pain distal to the area of TP. Snapping of the TP spot usually causes a local twitching of the muscle, which is usually painful.

The snapping or pressure at the area of TP usually results in Travell's jump sign.[340] This jump sign may be in the form of jumping off the examination table, crying out, wincing, or a guarding type of reflex.

The twitch response of Travell[340] is in the form of a transient contraction of the muscle under the area of needle stimulation or snapping palpation of TP. Each muscle has its own typical trigger point (Figure 33).

CRANIOFACIAL MUSCLES TRIGGER POINTS

The temporalis muscle has a trigger point mainly above the zygoma and close to TMJ. The sternocleidomastoid muscle causes referred pain to the occipital frontal region, and the TP is mainly over the sternal or clavicular heads of the muscle (Figure 22).

The upper and lower trapezius muscles are some of the most common areas of TP. Trigger point in the lower trapezius muscle results in pain over the shoulder or suboccipital region of the cervical paraspinal muscles, and injection in the lower trapezius area relieves this pain (Figure 22).

This lower trapezius muscle referred pain is quite common in cervical spine injuries and in RSD involving the upper extremity and shoulder. It explains why patients with cervical spine injuries complain of pain in T5, T6, and T7 paraspinal muscles on the same side (Figure 22).

The upper trapezius muscle has referred pain to the occipital and anterior, temporal, and frontal regions. Again, injection of the upper trapezius muscle results in good relief of pain. The masseteric muscle trigger point is quite commonly seen in TMJ disease, and injection of the masseteric muscle results in good relief (Figure 22).

CERVICAL SPINE TRIGGER POINTS

The trigger points as a result of neck injuries are usually present in the trapezius muscle as well as in the semispinalis cervicis, which causes occipital pain, and multifidi, which causes suboccipital pain. The splenius cervicis causes referred pain to the cervical paraspinal muscle region as well as the supraorbital region of the forehead.

SHOULDER AREA TRIGGER POINTS

The teres major trigger point injection relieves shoulder pain. So does the teres minor injection. The levator scapulae injection relieves pain in the cervical paraspinal region as well as in the shoulder area. The supra and infraspinatus injection as well as subscapularis injection also relieves pain in the shoulder region.

One common trigger point area is the cervical articular facet joint. Nerve block and injection of Depo-Medrol® relieves the headache (C2-4 level), shoulder pain (C4-6 level), and arms and hand pain (C5-T$_1$ level).

UPPER EXTREMITIES TRIGGER POINTS

Trigger point injection of the brachialis muscle relieves pain at the base of the thumb. The deltoid trigger point injection relieves pain in the shoulder. Trigger point injection in triceps muscle relieves pain in the elbow and fourth and fifth fingers of the hand. Trigger point injection of the extensor muscles of the forearm relieves pain in the wrist and dorsum of the hand.

Injecton of palmaris longus relieves pain in the palm of the hand.

Trigger point injection of the S1 level of paraspinal muscles relieves pain in the lumbar spine region as well as in the gluteal region.

TPI of the external oblique muscle relieves pain in the groin and epigastric region (Figure 22).

LOWER EXTREMITIES TRIGGER POINTS

Injection of the adductor muscles relieves pain in the groin and quadriceps region. TPI over the greater trochanteric region relieves pain in the lateral aspect of the thigh and lateral aspect of the legs below the knee.

Injection of the vastus intermedius relieves pain in the quadriceps region. Injection of the gluteus minimus results in relief of pain in the posterior aspect of the thigh and the leg and injection of the gluteus maximus relieves pain in the gluteal fold.

Injection of the tibialis TP injection relieves pain over the big toe, and injections of the soleus and gastrocnemius relieve pain over the heel and plantar aspect of the foot. Injection of the extensor digitorum longus relieves pain in the dorsum of the foot and injection of the peroneus longus and brevis relieves pain over the lateral aspect of the ankle and the foot (Figure 22).

TPI is effective if it is done with normal saline, xylocaine, or steroids. It has been shown that even insertion of a needle and irritation of the TP often times breaks down the vicious circle of vasoconstriction and helps the patient.

Injection with Depo-Medrol® is quite helpful as long as the injection does not cause leakage of the medication into the basal membrane of the dermis. Such an infiltration causes disruption of the melanin formation both locally and in referred areas distally. It can be quite upsetting for the patient because of the skin discoloration.

CLINICAL SIGNIFICANCE OF TRIGGER POINT

Any of the trigger points mentioned above has been referred to as "myofascial pain syndrome". This is unfortunate because it automatically deprives the patient of proper and effective treatments such as TPI or more effectively, articular facet joint nerve block and Depo-Medrol® injection.

The term has been so abused that whenever it appears in a report it implies that the patient does not have a disc herniation but has some vague problem.

In dealing with chronic pain,[306] the pain in the cervical and lumbar spine regions and the upper and lower extremities is caused by disc herniation in only one fourth the cases. The other three fourths are classified in all kinds of vague terminology, which does not help in either diagnosis or treatment of the patient.

The terminology should be limited to exact findings, i.e., either trigger point or localized injury to muscles, articular facets, skin lesion, etc. In this situation, thermography may be helpful in the diagnosis of soft tissue injuries.[409,410] The typical findings of thermography in soft tissue injuries are usually a localized area of decreased or increased temperature somewhere around 3 to 10 mm in diameter and frequently disc shaped (Figures 2a and 3). It should be at least 1–2°C below or above circumambient temperature of the surrounding area.[97,98]

It is quite common to see a cold zone in trigger point areas. A cold zone does not necessarily refer to a temporal factor — such as chronic lesions — but the cold zone is just as likely to develop in selected areas innervated by the sympathetic nerves resulting in vasoconstriction in a short period of time.

COLD SPOTS
The trigger point is usually a cold spot caused by subcutaneous reflex vasoconstriction due to referred pain. Occasionally the trigger point may be warmer than the surrounding skin (Figures 2a, 2b, and 3).

What determines whether the trigger point area is hot or cold is the interaction of multiple factors outlined above. For example, if there is a partial irritation of sympathetic nerves in the area of the trigger point, then the trigger point is going to be cold because of vasoconstriction.

Whether trigger point is a hot or cold spot, the injection of antiinflammatory medications such as Depo Medrol® causes marked relief of pain both in the trigger point area as well as in the area of the original source of nerve irritation.

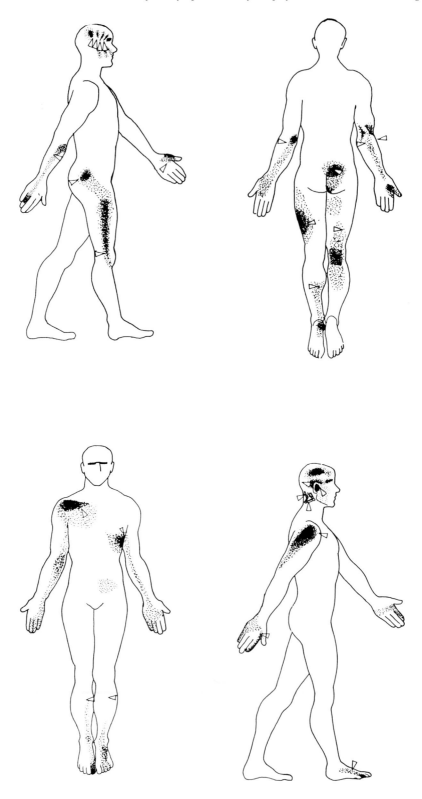

FIGURE 22. Trigger points as manifestations of referred pain.[376,377]

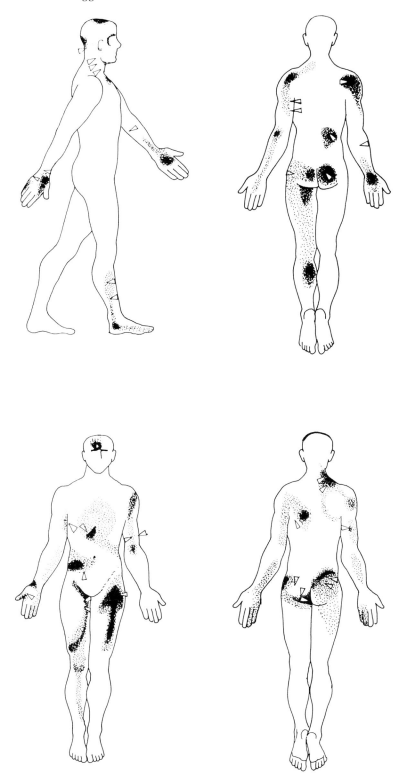

FIGURE 22b.

TABLE 11
Trigger Point

Results in
    Peripheral formation of substance P, norepinephrine, and vasoconstriction
    Chronic repetitive chemical injury commonly results in reflex focal vasoconstriction (cold spot)
    In rare cases, the longstanding vasoconstriction reflex is replaced by a decompensated focal vasodilation
    forming a "hot spot"

TRIGGER POINT INJECTION

As the trigger point is usually cold, pressure should be applied to reproduce the pain. With pressure, pain chemicals, such as substance P or lactic acid, are released subcutaneously, and immediately the trigger point becomes red. The injection with Depo-Medrol® should be deep, not subcutaneous. If the steroid is injected at the basement membrane of the skin, melanin is destroyed, and the patient develops whitish discoloration of the skin.

In the case of ephaptic RSD it is dangerous and quite painful to the patient to inject the area of scarring of axonal electric short (such as in the dorsum of the hand, dorsum of the foot, or around the knee). On the other hand, when such an area of ephaptic dystrophy causes a referred trigger point, hot or cold (usually cold), the injection of this area causes significant relief on the basis of Sherrington's principle of internuncial pools in the substantia nigra.[573]

For example, ephaptic migraine vascular headache as a referred pain may be secondary to injury of the articular facets of the third or fourth cervical vertebrae and can be relieved by repetitive injections of the articular facet trigger point (Figures 16 and 22). Such patients are mistakenly diagnosed with migraine headaches.

In the above-mentioned example, the patient's trigger point may be as far away as the area of the sternomastoid muscle or the area of the mid or upper thoracic paraspinal muscles.

As long as the topical scarred area of the ephaptic nerve damage is not injected, the trigger point injection will cause a significant reduction in the patient's pain. (See also Chapter 12 under "Trigger Point Injection".)

9

Etiology of RSD

Contrary to general impression, trauma is not at the top of the list in the etiology of RSD (Table 12). Other diseases are more likely to be complicated by RSD. The factors that contribute to the development of RSD in different illnesses are

1. Chemical, e.g., chemical burns are quite frequently accompanied by RSD.
2. Anatomical, such as disruption of myelin in diabetic neuropathy.
3. Vascular, such as disturbance of microcirculation in diabetic neuropathy.
4. Electrical, such as causalgia, electrical injuries, bullet injuries, sharp object injuries.
5. Infection, e.g., postherpetic neuralgia.
6. Demyelination, multiple sclerosis and diabetes.
7. Hyperpathic pain generated by diseases such as coronary artery insufficiency and heart attacks that result in shoulder-hand syndrome.

Chemical burns are at the top of the frequency list, followed by postherpetic neuralgia, electrical injuries, and diabetes (Table 12).

CERVICAL SPINE AND RSD

Cervical spine pathology is quite frequently accompanied by RSD. The frequent association of RSD with cervical spine pathology is the result of the fact that vertebral arteries are accompanied by rich plexus of sympathetic nerve fibers. As a result, the traumatic spondylotic type of pathology in the cervical spine causes involvement of the sympathetic system with secondary complex manifestations of dizziness, chest wall pain, etc. (Figure 23).

In addition, trauma to the cervical spine results in referred pain in the distribution of the trigeminal nerve as well as referred pain to the upper thoracic spine region (Figures 16 and 23).

Barré and Lieou in 1926[18] pointed to cervical spine pathology causing sympathetic dysfunction (Barré-Lieou syndrome). Unfortunately, the role of cervical spine pathology in RSD has been recognized by few clinicians.

The complex anatomical structures of the cervical spine is richly innervated by the sympathetic nervous system (Figure 23).

As recognized by Barré in 1928,[18] the sympathetic nerves traverse through the different structures of the cervical spine. The deep sympathetic plexus surrounding the vertebral arteries plays a major role in the development of vertigo, blurring of vision, and ataxia secondary to cervical spine pathology (Figure 23).

TABLE 12
Etiology of RSD

Etiology of RSD	RSD/total[a]	Percent
Chemical burns (causalgia)	4/5	80
Postherpetic (neuralgia) (face, eye, trunk)	31/39	79
Electrical injuries (causalgia)	33/42	72
Spinal cord tumor	4/17	57
Diabetic neuropathy[b] (neuropathic pain)	18/54	33
TMJ disease	3/11	27
Posttraumatic	101/482	21
Cervical spondylosis	42/328	12
Multiple sclerosis	20/182	11
Atypical facial pain		(2.4)
Trigeminal neuralgia		(4.5)
Extremities RSD		(3)
Dysautonomic attacks		(1)
Diarrhea		
Coronary artery disease	6/69	9
Stroke	18/223	8
Thalamic infarct with thalamic pain, RSD of disuse in spastic extremity		

[a] Incidence of RSD was determined with the help of thermography. To estimate the figures without the use of thermography, divide by 4.
[b] Stewart et al.[58] found sympathetic involvement in 80% of such patients.

The sympathetic nerves innervating the different structures in the cervical spine region terminate in different end organs with a variety of symptomatologies as the manifestation of cervical spine disease (Figure 23).

CERVICAL SPONDYLOSIS

One common illness that frequently is misdiagnosed or undiagnosed is cervical spondylosis. Cervical spondylosis due to aging, degenerative changes, and dehydration of the disc spaces in the cervical spine results in a complex clinical picture.

Usually cervical spondylosis is asymptomatic. It is not at all unusual to see all forms of osteophytes, desiccated disc spaces, narrowed disc spaces, and other degenerative changes in cervical spine X-rays of people who are 40 to 45 years old. Spondylosis should *not* be called arthritis; there is no inflammation. It is nature's defense against drying up (desiccation) of joints and disc spaces due to aging. It usually does not cause any pain unless some form of trauma disrupts nature's fine balance.

Certain diseases that accelerate aging make the patient more susceptible to the development of cervical spondylosis. These consist of alcohol abuse, which causes dehydration of the disc spaces, excessive cigarette smoking, oophorectomy with resultant early osteoporosis and bone degeneration, and repeated traumas (e.g., playing football, hard labor).

Cervical spondylosis is usually asymptomatic. The osteophytes form a partial internal brace and limit the range of motion of the cervical spine to protect the vertebrae and other anatomical structures from undergoing further damage in a patient who has dehydrated disc spaces.

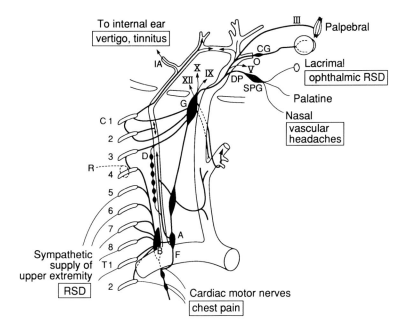

FIGURE 23. Cervical sympathetic system and related symptoms.

When this natural defense becomes decompensated, a complex clinical picture develops encompassing a range of symptoms as common as headache and dizziness, RSD, and shoulder-hand syndrome, and as rare as hemifacial spasm and blepharospasm (Table 13).

TREATMENT OF CERVICAL SPONDYLOSIS

Cervical spondylosis is only matched by diabetes and syphilis as the "master immitators" in neurology. When dealing with headache, dizziness, shoulder pain, arm pain, or unexplained chest pain, cervical spondylosis should be considered at the top of the list of differential diagnosis.

Even when diagnosed, it is called arthritis, which it is not. Arthritis means inflammation. Spondylosis is not due to inflammation but is due to old trauma or wear and tear of life: osteophyte formation that is usually trauma.

By improperly calling it arthritis, the patient is unnecessarily exposed to strong antiinflammatory medications with serious side effects. Proper diagnosis and terminology result in successful treatment with traction, heat, and massage.

The schedule of treatment for cervical spondylosis is outlined in Table 14.

Table 14 summarizing the various symptoms of cervical spondylosis would be longer and more complex if other rare symptoms of cervical spondylosis were included.

When dealing with typical headache, face pain, or dizziness, one should consider cervical spine pathology. In such conditions, MRI and CT scan of the head are normal, but the cervical spine is ignored as the cause.

Tests that provide the most accurate diagnosis of cervical spine pathology consist of proper cervical spine X-rays, MRI, EMG, evoked potentials, especially BAER for dizziness, and thermography when RSD is suspected. The thermography should include not only the head and face area but the posterior cervical spine region as well as upper extremities.

The correct diagnosis of such complex neurologic manifestations is not simply an academic exercise.

Practically all the complex symptoms outlined in Table 13 show excellent response to treatment with physiotherapy, especially traction, moist heat, as well as muscle relaxants.

TABLE 13
Symptoms of Cervical Spondylosis

Symptoms of spondylosis	Disease mistaken for
Vertigo secondary to pressure on vertebral artery	Meniere's disease
	Inner ear disease
RSD with spasm around the shoulder girdle and secondary bursitis ligament injury	Bursitis
	Rotator cuff injury
	Shoulder ligament injury
	Shouder-hand syndrome
Pain and RSD down the hands and elbow	Carpal tunnel syndrome
	Tardy ulnar palsy and unnecessary surgery
Referred pain to pectoralis trapezius scalene areas	Thoracic outlet syndrome: thoracic outlet syndrome rarely is symptomatic. Even then, it is usually caused by scalenus anticus spasm due to RSD and chronic pain
Tremor, dystonia	Familial essential tremor
	Dystonia
Hemifacial spasm and blepharospasm as referred spasm (rare)	Essential blepharospasm improperly treated with surgery or botulinum toxin injection
Vascular headaches	Migraine
Occipital neuralgia	Idiopathic occipital neuralgia
	Occipital nerve section has disastrous results
Ophthalmic nerve referred pain to forehead	Trigeminal neuralgia treated with unnecessary surgery
Vertebral basilar artery insufficiency (VBI)	Stroke
	Bell's palsy
	Meniere's disease
	Inner ear disease
	Idiopathic ataxia, etc.
Chest pain	Coronary artery disease
	Angina pectoris

TABLE 14
Management of Cervical Spondylosis[a]

Traction both at home and at physiotherapy department. The traction should be done on a daily basis at home as well as 2 to 3 times a week at the physiotherapy department
Moist heat
Muscle relaxants [e.g., baclofen (Lioresol), carisoprodol (Soma), cyclobenzapine (Flexeril)]
Massage, ultrasound
Trigger point injections
In severe cases, antiinflammatory medications

[a] The same treatments and principles apply to chronic cervical spine injury.

CHRONIC CERVICAL SPINE INJURY

In patients who suffer from intractable migraine headaches especially among the younger generation in children and teenagers, proper cervical spine examination reveals the source of the severe migraine vascular headaches in the cervical spine region.

Aiming the treatment at cervical spine pathology is quite helpful in controlling such headaches.

The diagnosis is quite difficult because of the fact that the same trauma that has caused chronic cervical spine injury also quite frequently has caused simultaneous head injury and amnesia. As a result, the patient does not remember the accident.

One common situation is when a child falls off a swing at the school grounds or is involved in a car accident and is unconscious for a few seconds, has some headache, neck pain, and vomiting for a few days, and then everything clears up. The problem reappears as severe vascular headache years later. In such patients, careful evaluation of cervical spine can discover the cervical spine pathology.

The amnesia from the head injury deprives the clinician of the history of trauma and makes the diagnosis more difficult. Hence, these patients are classified as "idiopathic" migraine.

SHERRINGTON'S PHENOMENON

As shown in Figure 16, Sherrington's[579] principle of overlapping pools at the substantia gelatinosa at the upper cervical spinal cord region explains the reason for referred pain to the face with resultant facial pain and headache and referred pain to the shoulder with resultant bursitis and shoulder-hand syndrome.

The c fibers carrying pain from the cervical spine region, especially from the C1 through C4 levels, enter the substantia gelatinosa and are superimposed by the sensory nerve fibers from the ophthalmic branch of the trigeminal nerve in the same area of the spinal cord.

As a result, the Sherrington pool stimulation of these sensory nerve fibers results in referred pain to the retroorbital region and frontal region of the face.

At the level of C4 substantia gelatinosa, the overlap of the nerves from the posterior cervical region with the nerves from the deltoid and pectoralis muscles results in referred pain to the shoulder and resultant muscle spasm and limitation of motion of the shoulder with secondary shoulder-hand syndrome and bursitis of the shoulder (Figure 16).

CERVICAL SPINE AND CHEST PAIN

In cervical spondylosis on the basis of the same Sherrington phenomenon, the pain may radiate to the chest wall and precordial region after stimulation of the cardiac plexus (Figure 23).

The pain in such patients is practically identical to coronary artery disease, and the patient may end up undergoing unnecessary coronary angiography and coronary bypass surgery.

Usually traction, moist heat, and muscle relaxants correct this condition, and in 11 patients who had such symptoms secondary to cervical spondylosis, only two required cervical fusion (one at the C3–4 and C4–5 level, and the other at the C4–5 level) with complete relief of neck pain.

TREMOR AND CERVICAL SPINE PATHOLOGY

Cervicogenic RSD in rare cases can cause tremor in the hand and forearm, and in some cases it can be severe enough to cause writer's cramp and illegible handwriting. This complication is more commonly seen after traumatic adjustment of the cervical spine.

Treatment of choice is the same as outlined for chest pain and cervicogenic RSD.

In two patients, we had to resort to cervical fusion to correct the tremor. In one case the tremor disappeared, and in the other case it was improved by at least 50%.

OTHER SYSTEMIC CAUSES OF RSD

Other less common causes of RSD consist of cancer, especially cancer of the lung with involvement of the apex.[264] RSD may in rare cases be the heralding symptoms of certain neurologic illnesses such as syringomyelia and Parkinson's disease.[75,359] It may complicate TMJ disease and vice versa.[232] More frequently it may be the initial manifestation of metabolic illnesses such as gout.[191]

RSD can be associated with a preexisting disease that has already been diagnosed such as diabetes (see Table 12) or may accompany psychiatric pathology such as chronic psychosis.[264]

At times hypnotics and tranquilizers not only aggravate RSD, but they may be etiologic factors in RSD after a minor trauma.[388]

The drugs that are more likely to be accompanied by RSD are the same drugs (alcohol, phenobarbital,[388] and benzodiazepines) that significantly affect temporal frontal lobes, and, as a result, predispose the patient to hyperpathia and allodynia.

IDIOPATHIC FORMS OF RSD

Aseptic necrosis of the hip and migratory osteolysis have been linked to RSD.[313] As is the case with almost all idiopathic illnesses, the reason the condition is idiopathic is because of either the failure to recognize the disease or the patient's reluctance to discuss the etiology, or the patient's amnesia regarding the original etiology (trauma).

Every time we deal with "idiopathic" disease in medicine, alcohol abuse should be considered as the cause.

ALCOHOL ABUSE AND RSD

The sympathetic nervous system is a most efficient system in thermal regulation. While recording the patient's movements during polysomnography, we have noted the patient reflexly and automatically responds to ambient temperature changes. When the temperature turns cooler, the sleeping patient reflexly reaches for a cover and protects the body against temperature loss.

As the room temperature increases, the patient automatically kicks off the covers and stimulates surface temperature loss.

This reflex temperature regulation is intact in sober individuals. When the ethanol intake increases over 120 ml within 4 hours prior to sleep, this temperature regulation becomes disrupted.

Excessive alcohol intake paralyzes temperature regulation and results in hypothermia when the patient is exposed to a cold environment.

Alcohol reduces the REM sleep. The same is true with barbiturates. On the other hand, certain antidepressants such as trazodone increase REM sleep time.[518] This may explain the beneficial effect of trazodone and the harmful effect of alcohol and barbiturates on RSD. By reducing the REM sleep, the patient is tired and depressed the next day due to poor quality of sleep. This causes a vicious circle of inactivity conducive to RSD.

The same alcohol abuse and head injury that are the major contributors of idiopathic migraine headache, idiopathic epilepsy, and idiopathic depression, they can also be the cause of idiopathic RSD. In alcohol abuse patients and head injury patients, the following forms of RSD may be present.

Focal osteoporosis[330-334] is the transient type of focal regional osteoporosis. This condition may be seen in an elderly person who may have had a fall and may not remember it. The fall may have caused injury to the hip or to the hand or foot and then may spontaneously clear up.

Usually what has seemed to be an idiopathic form of RSD quite frequently has frontal temporal lobe dysfunction as the etiologic factor. This frontal temporal lobe dysfunction can be due to trauma or drugs such as alcohol, barbiturates, and other CNS depressants.

In this regard, diagnostic tests such as PET scanning or topographic brain mapping may be the only diagnostic link and evidence between the idiopathic RSD and the cause of this condition.

The involvement of the highest centers of the brain (frontal lobes and limbic system) is quite common in advanced stages of RSD (Stage IV).

As a matter of fact, the following would be a better categorization of RSD.

1.   Early reflex sympathetic dysfunction
2.   Subacute reflex sympathetic dystrophy

3. Advanced reflex sympathetic atrophy
4. Chronic Stage IV of reflex sympathetic dystrophy and atrophy with the main manifestation of neuropsychiatric cerebral dysfunction

The main manifestations of the neuropsychiatric cerebral dysfunction are phobia, depression, extremely low threshold for pain, tendency for suicide, marked movement disorders in the form of spasticity, weakness of extremity, tremor and dystonia, and episodic agitated behavior interspersed with schizoaffective behavior.

The depressive and schizoaffective behaviors can alternate in the same patient due to bilateral limbic system and frontal lobe involvement in Stage IV advanced RSD. Such posttraumatic manifestations of chronic pain can be present in RSD, electrical injuries, and head injuries.[242]

In Stage IV of RSD, the condition can be severe enough that the patient may require morphine pump. Otherwise, in rare cases may require electroshock treatment to prevent a suicidal attempt.

Chronic pain, chronic complications of head injuries, RSD, chemical burn, and electrical injuries are explicit models of organic damages manifesting themselves as practically pure psychiatric illnesses. Even more common than the above examples and usually accompanied by some of the above examples is the case of alcoholism.

Alcoholism is the best kept secret in medicine when studying subjects such as hypertension, diabetes, pancreatitis, peptic ulcer, nutritional neuropathy, cirrhosis, and Gilles de la Tourette syndrome.[480] The majority of these patients are children of alcoholics.[480] Fetal alcohol syndrome is the number one cause of retardation[481] and many other illnesses (e.g., childhood schizophrenia and autism).

Doctors are reluctant to delve into the history of alcoholism. Not infrequently, blaming the patient for drinking causes such hostility on the side of the patient that the doctor has a fear of a malpractice suit. It is quite easy for the alcoholic to find another doctor who would use a dual diagnosis name (as outlined above) for the patient's addiction and would tell the patient that the condition has nothing to do with alcoholism. This would prompt the alcoholic to start a malpractice suit against the first doctor. In the case of RSD when every aggressive form of treatment fails, one should suspect a closet drinker using alcohol as an analgesic. Such patients are typically labeled idiopathic causalgia.

It is impossible to manage the problem of RSD without addressing the problem of the patient being an undiagnosed alcoholic. Of the drug abuses in society, alcohol is third in incidence, trailing food and cigarettes.

Alcohol as the "gate" drug is most addictive due to its multiple manipulative effects on the brain.

1. Alcohol simultaneously stimulates (in small doses) and destroys (in large doses) the dopamine, serotonin, endorphin, BZ, GABA, and other neurotransmitters (Figure 28). Both alcohol and cocaine accelerate the breakdown of dopamine presynaptically. These two drugs have identical effect on synapse and ion channels:

    a. Small doses of alcohol go through dopamine ion channels: stimulant effect of alcohol.
    b. Moderate doses of alcohol: GABA channels open: tranquility.
    c. Large doses of alcohol: kainate and quisqualate channels become flooded: coma and death.

2. Alcohol kills the nerves that generate the essential neurotransmitters and leaves the brain dependent on outside sources for chemicals simulating such neurotransmitters (Figure 28).

3.   Alcohol disrupts the function of the large synaptic transfer polypeptide protein[479] that is responsible for the transfer and replenishment of the neurotransmitters such as serotonin, dopamine, and GABA (Figure 28).
4.   Alcohol is an unstable and volatile source of energy that is rapidly utilized by the nerve cells. In this regard, alcohol becomes addictive just like sugar becomes addictive for an already defective malnourished and damaged brain.
5.   As alcohol disrupts the absorption and utilization of coenzymes and vitamins, the brain must rely on the utilization of rapidly burning carbohydrates such as sugar (sucrose) and alcohol. In this process, self-perpetuating malnutrition, damage, and destruction ensue.
6.   Alcohol coagulates the proteins and disrupts the function of coenzymes, vitamins, and hormones and deprives the brain of the anabolic reconstruction of the partially damaged nerve cells. It accelerates the aging and destruction of the CNS. The brain of an alcoholic at age 37 is identical to the brain of a nondrinker at the age of 67 when viewed on a CT scan or MRI test.
7.   A patient suffering from RSD, low pain threshold, and depression cannot afford the destructive effect of any of the three major categories of addictive drugs, i.e., alcohol, narcotics, or cocaine (Figure 28).
     (See also Chapter 11 under "Avoidance of Alcohol".)

INTERCOSTAL RSD

In the case of intercostal RSD, the two most common etiologies are herpes zooster and diabetes. At times herpes zooster[335] may cause recurrence of pain without skin eruption, and in this situation thermography may be quite helpful in identifying such attacks causing painful RSD. Treatment with large doses of acyclovir in such patients results in good control of pain. Capsaicin applied topically is quite helpful in the acute stage of the illness. Acyclovir at 1600–2400 mg a day given for 2 to 3 months provides excellent relief of pain and control of the illness. Acyclovir treatment of 1–2 weeks is apt to fail because of the long half-life of herpes virus.

As is the case with all other RSD patients, the earlier the diagnosis, the more successful is the treatment. In subacute stages, treatment with steroids such as dexamethasone and prednisone should be replaced with ACTH therapy.

SPINAL CORD RSD

Injury to the spinal cord[482] results in sympathetic hyperreflexia. This is in the form of vasoconstriction, piloerection, hypothermia, and sweating in the distal portion of the spinal cord injury. Systemic hypertension, bradycardia, and cardiac arrythmias are not uncommon.

RSD is frequently a complication and manifestation of spinal cord pathology — trauma (Figure 24) or tumor (Table 15). One bedside sign of spinal cord pathology is the skin's response to gentle superficial scratching with a safety pin. Distal to the level of spinal cord pathology there is a hyperactive vasoconstrictive response to the superficial scratching. In total paraplegia, there is a decompensated vasodilation.

Traumatic myelopathy (Figure 24) can be complicated with RSD in different degrees.

Incomplete lesions of the spinal cord are more likely to be complicated with RSD. Even after recovery from partial lesions of the spinal cord, severe pain may appear as a sign of RSD, which may be relieved by sympathectomy.[471]

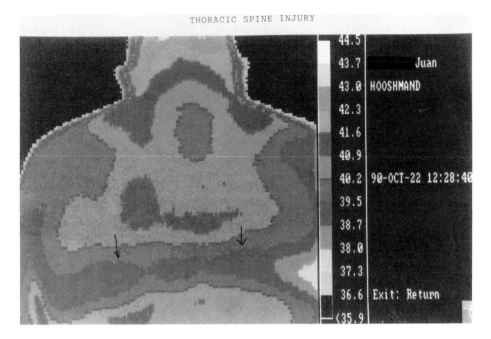

FIGURE 24. Thoracic spine injury with chest wall pain and neurogenic bladder. X-rays and MRI were normal. Thermography shows T5–6 nerve roots injury. Somatosensory evoked potentials were abnormal pointing to spinal cord injury. See also color plates following page 42.

TABLE 15
Spinal Cord Pathology

RSD is a common manifestation of
  Spinal cord injury (Figure 25)
  MS involving spinal cord
  Spinal cord tumors
  Syrinx

ELECTRICAL INJURIES

In our experience of over 100 patients suffering from electrical injuries referred to our clinic from differents parts of the country, 42 patients had comprehensive extensive studies, both anatomical and physiological.

The rest of the patients had the majority of their studies done in other centers, and they are not included in this series of 42 patients being reported because there was not a complete battery of anatomical tests (MRI or CT), neuropsychometric tests (Halstead-Reitan or Luria-Nebraska), and neurophysiologic tests (evoked potentials and topographic brain mapping).

The following is a summary of the stereotypical clinical findings on electrical injuries. Thirty-three of 42 patients suffered from RSD. The treatment for the patients suffering from RSD secondary to causalgic pain of electrical contact was quite difficult and taxing to the clinician and to the patient.

As with other forms of RSD, the disease is classified into four stages.

Stage I: On the Scene of the Accident

1. No-let-go phenomenon. This was present in practically every patient except for the ones who had exposure to electricity to areas that could not undergo gripping of the hand, such as contact with the foot or dorsum of the forearm (Figure 5a). No-let-go phenomenon means the electrical stimulation causes flexor spasm of the muscles, not allowing the victim to let go of the electrical source.
2. Ipsilateral extremity burn, eschar, and neurosensory damage. The same phenomenon to a lesser extent is present in the contralateral extremity — exit point of the electricity. The lesion specifically involves c fiber nerves and nerves around the arterioles (sympathetic nerve fibers) with ephapse in c fibers. As a result, the patient has severe pain in the involved areas, and the pain extends far beyond the eschar region.
3. The body is usually thrown away from the source of electricity in one massive myoclonic jerk. This results in falling from a ladder or other heights with secondary injuries.
4. Tonic and at times tonic clonic seizures of brief duration, followed by a brief loss of consciousness.
5. Cardiac arrhythmias and brief cardiac arrest with good response to resuscitation, followed by typical autonomic dysfunction in the form of abnormal cardiac rhythm, fluctuating blood pressure, and abdominal and chest pains. Attacks of apnea are quite frequent.
6. Blisters over the fingers, acute RSD of extremity, blisters and reddish discoloration over the contralateral exit point, as well as blisters and reddish discolorations over the anterior chest wall at T4 through T6 levels, which are the points of entrance of electricity through vascular and sympathetic fibers to the spinal cord (Figure 4d).

Stage II: Hospitalization

1. The patient is quite drowsy and at times confused and tired.
2. Labile vital signs in the first 24 hours, prolonged PQ, deep Q, irregular PQ interval, and arhythmias on EKG. Orthostatic hypotension is quite common at this stage, resulting in syncopal attack when the patient tries to get up and walk.
3. Akinetic attacks. Usually myoclonic seizures are less frequent at this stage, and they are more likely to develop in Stages III or IV.
4. Vertigo and tinnitus, which can be quite intractable, lasting for months to years.
5. Painful extremities at the points of entrance and exit, eschars of different degrees, and RSD.
6. Sensory loss over the trunk distal to the T4 through T6 entrance of electricity to the spinal cord. This sensory loss is usually asymmetrical, and the patient usually develops a partial Brown-Sequard syndrome.
    This aspect of the examination should be checked on every patient. This is the most frequently overlooked and underdiagnosed sign of electrical injuries.
    This sign of spinal cord injury explains the reason for the patient having myoclonic and akinetic seizures too deep to be recorded on EEG.
    This is practically pathognomic and was present in every patient.
7. Frontal lobe dysfunction: tremor, positive snout reflex, masked fascies, irritability, and poor judgment were present in over 50% of the patients.

Stage III: First Few Weeks to Months after the Accident

1. Extremities pain, hyperpathia, and allodynia were present in 29 of 42 patients.
2. Akinetic or myoclonic seizures were present in 28 of 42 patients.
3. Anxiety, agitation, phobia, irritability.
4. Labile neurovascular symptoms and signs:
    a. Cardiac arrhythmias
    b. RSD
    c. Labile blood pressure, orthostatic hypotension
    d. Abdominal cramps
    e. Diarrhea
    f. Noncardiac origin chest wall pain usually due to sympathetic nerve injury (Figures 4d and 4e).
5. Poor recall, poor recent memory.
6. Depression and secondary insomnia were present in 28 of 42 patients.
7. Frontal lobe dysfunction, irritability, tremor, poor judgment, poor tolerance, and fatigue.

Stage IV: Over 6 Months

1. Loss of job (over 50% of the patients).
2. Loss of spouse, severe marital interpersonal strain (over 50% of patients).
3. Vertigo and tinnitus in one-third of patients.
4. Severe depression or schizoeffective withdrawal, anxiety, phobia in over three-fourths of the patients.
5. Akinetic and myoclonic seizures.
6. Poor recall and recent memory in over 60% of the patients.
7. Painful extremity (chronic pain) in over 30% of the patients.
8. RSD in 33 of 42 patients.
9. Impotence, neurogenic bladder, abdominal cramps, and chronic tremor.

DIAGNOSTIC TESTS FOR ELECTRICAL INJURIES

1. Anatomical tests, i.e., MRI or CT scans are normal.
2. Physiological tests:
    a. EEG usually is normal: 7 (14%) patients had sharp transients, and 4 (9%) had epileptiform discharges in the temporal frontal regions.
    b. EKG abnormal in Stages I and II in over 50% of the patients. The EKG subsequently reverted to normal.
    c. Thermography was abnormal in 33 of 42 patients, showing different degrees of RSD (Figures 4d, 4e, and 25).
    d. Evoked potentials.
        i.   Visual evoked potentials are usually nondiagnostic.
        ii. Baer showed abnormalities in interpeaks I–III in 30 of 42 patients and in 21 of 42 patients in stage IV.
        iii. SSEP was abnormal in 39 of 42 patients in Stages I–III and 27 of 42 in Stage IV.
    e. Topographic brain mapping was abnormal in 28 of 42 patients in Stages III and IV. None was done in Stages I and II.

The low percentage of EEG abnormality may be due to (1) involvement of deep structures, and (2) tests done in late (chronic) stages of the disease.

The abnormality on topographic brain mapping is usually in the form of frontal temporal asymmetry and suppression of background, which was bilateral in 22 of 28 brain mappings.

In two patients, α dislocation was noted. This phenomenon refers to the fact that the α frequency power spectrum has shifted from the occipital lobes to the frontal lobes. These patients had suffered from prolonged coma after the electrical injury. They suffered from a marked frontal lobe dysfunction as mentioned above.

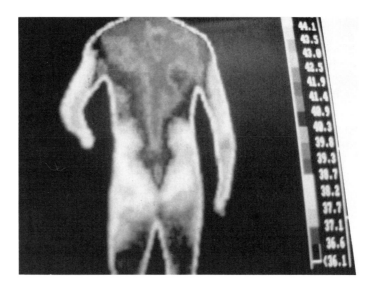

FIGURE 25. Multiple peripheral and central nervous system electrical injuries. RSD in involved extremities. Thoracic spinal cord injury at point of electrical entrance through C-fibers (sympathetic nerves) (also see Figures 4d–4f). Brain stem dysfunction (vertigo with abnormal evoked potentials). Limbic system dysfunctions: depression, memory loss, poor judgment, abnormal topographic brain mapping as well as abnormal Halstead-Reitan test. See also color plates following page 42.

The only other condition that causes α dislocation on brain mapping is rare severe head injuries or cerebral anoxia, which shows "α coma" on the EEG as well.

The electrical injury causes CNS damage and follows the path of least resistance, which is the c fibers and the sympathetic nerve fibers surrounding the arteries to the thoracic spinal cord. The damage ascends up and down to the lower portion of the spinal cord in the final pathways of the nociceptive c fibers (Figures 4d–f, 25, and Table 14).

DIFFERENTIAL DIAGNOSIS OF RSD

DISEASES MISTAKEN FOR RSD

1. Scleroderma. Thermography helps differentiate it from RSD. Thermography shows clearly the delineated line of demarkation between cold fingers and warm palm of the hand in scleroderma. This is in contrast to the glove type of cold upper extremity in RSD, a selective nerve involvement in nerve root injuries (Figure 26).
2. Occlusive peripheral arterial disease. Doppler ultrasound studies as well as absence of peripheral pulse are helpful in differentiating this condition from RSD.
3. Spinal cord tumors, syringomelia, and contusion of spinal cord are almost invariably associated with RSD. In so-called idiopathic RSD, the above conditions need to be ruled out.
4. Raynaud's syndrome (Raynaud, 1862)[476a] is vascular dysfunction of the extremities, which is usually benign. This prognostic feature separates it from more severe forms of RSD.

The condition is a good example of the central origin of sympathetic dysfunction. The local vasoconstrictor reflex that is absent in peripheral nerve damages such as diabetic neuropathy[477a]

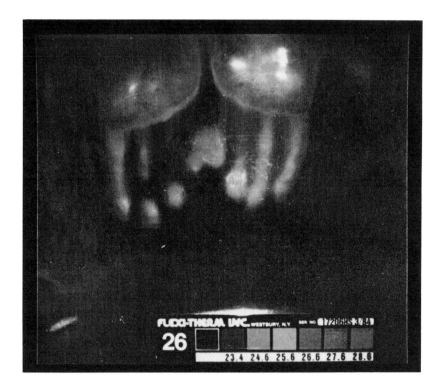

FIGURE 26. Scleroderma may be mistaken for RSD. Thermography easily differentiates it: the hypothermia is limited to fingers only and spares the palm of the hand. See also color plates following page 42.

stays intact in Raynaud's phenomenon. On the other hand, vasoconstrictive responses to sitting or standing are increased in Raynaud's phenomenon.[478a]

In our experience with 26 consecutive cases of Raynaud's phenomenon, migraine headache was a concomitant complication in 17 patients. This high incidence of migraine headaches also suggests a central origin of the vascular dysfunction.

RSD MISTAKEN FOR OTHER DISEASES

One aspect of efferent dysfunction of RSD is spasm in the shoulder girdle muscles, pectoralis muscles, and scalenus muscles. The latter group of muscles undergoing spasm cause the clinical picture of thoracic outlet syndrome.

1. Thoracic outlet syndrome. As is the case with cervical disc herniation, cervical nerve roots contusion, cervical spondylosis, and soft tissue injuries to the cervical spine region, RSD patients are quite frequently diagnosed with thoracic outlet syndrome. Unnecessary surgery for such patients is frought with disastrous results.
    Usually facial injury causes referred pain to the C3 and C4 substantia gelatinosa gray matter of the spinal cord. This in turn causes spasm over deltoid and scalenus muscles. The end result is not only TMJ disease, but shoulder-hand syndrome and thoracic outlet syndrome. The combination of any two of the above three conditions points to RSD as the etiology. Obviously surgery for any of the above conditions produces disastrous results.
2. Entrapment neuropathies such as carpal tunnel syndrome and tardy ulnar palsy are frequently mistaken diagnoses for RSD. Surgery in such cases is apt to aggravate the RSD, which has gone undiagnosed (Figure 17).

3.   Rotator cuff injury or tear of the shoulder. It is not unusual to see a patient suffering from advanced RSD who has undergone multiple surgical procedures from the hand all the way to the shoulder with mistaken diagnoses of carpal tunnel syndrome, tardy ulnar palsy, and rotator cuff injury. Each one of the above surgical procedures cumulatively aggravates the RSD.

4.   Knee injuries. It is not uncommon for the patient to sustain a blunt injury to the anterolateral aspect of the knee. This can cause RSD with afferent (pain) and efferent (limitation of motion of knee) complications. The arthroscopy done on such knee injury is "the straw that breaks the camel's back" and causes severe aggravation of RSD.

TABLE 16
Final Clinical Diagnosis in 100 Patients
Diagnosed as Multiple Sclerosis on
MRI (1985–1991)

Diagnosis	Number
Multiple sclerosis	78
Old head injuries	12
Congenital or early infancy defect(s)	4
Lyme disease	2
HTLV infection	1
Vasculitis (neurosyphilis)	1
Cause unknown (not multiple scleroris)	2
	100

10

Diagnosis of RSD

> "The key to successful management of RSD
> is early diagnosis (within first 6 months)."
>
> Poplawski et al.[280]

The peripheral nervous system has three main neurophysiologic features that can be evaluated independently: sensory, autonomic, and motor features — "SAM" — as termed by Dr. J. Green (in lectures given regarding chronic pain). The sensory function is best examined clinically and with the help of SSEP,[93,391] the autonomic system is best evaluated by thermography,[293] and the motor system is best evaluated by EMG.

RSD is diagnosed by different methods: (1) clinical, (2) bone scan, (3) skin conductance response, (4) capillary blood cell velocity (CBV), laser doppler fluxmetry (LDF), and (5) thermography, and (6) quantitative sweat autonomic response test (QSART).

CLINICAL TESTS

This is done by observation, palpation, and examination of the extremity. This is quite a limited method, and it is mainly helpful in the diagnosis of advanced second and third stages of RSD, hence, the reason for early medical literature emphasizing the rare cases of causalgia.

In addition to observation of color changes, edema, tremor, and spasticity, the following tests should be done: orthostatic BP tests, heart rate response to deep breathing and tilt test, Valsalva's maneuver, and effects of above procedures on pulse and BP.

Clinical examination is quite informative in the diagnosis of trigger points as the manifestation of RSD. Careful bedside examination identifies cervical spine pathology as the source of craniocervical RSD with secondary vascular headache.

In reflex sympathetic dysfunction (RSD 1), early vasoconstriction, pain, discomfort, hyperhydrosis (excessive sweating), and mild tenderness to touch are the main clinical features of the disease.

The clinical examination becomes more informative in Stages II–IV of RSD.

MEASUREMENT OF PAIN

1. **Clinical measurement**. Pain contrary to its **legal definition is *not* subjective**. An acute **myocardial infarction** chest pain is quite objective: **grayish color of skin, diffuse sweating, shock,** etc.

The more subtle form of pain may be measured as follows:

The clinical measurement has been outlined in detail by Davidoff et al.[73]

DAVIDOFF METHOD[73]

A measurement of joint pain of the hand and feet by palpation can be specified on a scale of 0 to +4: (0) no pain, (1) mild pain, (2) severe pain to deep palpation, (3) severe pain to mild palpation, and (4) hyperesthesia and hyperalgesia (the patient does not allow palpation).

2. Movement disorders. The pain of RSD is quite commonly and frequently accompanied by flexion deformity of elbow, hand, and joints. In addition, quite frequently it is accompanied by tremor or other movement disorders such as dystonia.

Frequently the pain is accompanied by hyperhydrosis and abnormal hair growth (cholinergic dysfunction).

3. Limb volume. Early in the course of RSD an asymmetrical increase and swelling of the limb volume occurs. The foot swelling measurement can be achieved by immersion of the foot into a five-gallon fish tank. Similar measurement can be made of the hand; and if the reading is difficult, the hand can be immersed up to the lateral malleolus in a 2-liter laboratory beaker. A foot is immersed to 6 cm up to approximately the distal edge of the lateral malleolus. An average of two to four trials can be made, and the results can be recorded. The same is done with the opposite limb.

Davidoff et al.[73] created the following formula, which helps measure the limb volume: volume of affected limb minus volume of unaffected limb results in a figure that is multiplied by 100 and divided by the volume of the unaffected limb. Any limb difference of more than 5% is considered by Davidoff et al. as abnormal.

4. Active and passive range of motion of the extremity can be measured by an inclinometer and goneometer, and compared with the opposite. It should be realized that RSD quite frequently tends to become bilateral and as a result it is best to compare the measurements with normal limb measurements of a control population rather than the opposite limb.

5. McGill Pain Questionnaire (MPQ)[219] yields informative results by the parameters of a pain rating index (PRI). This is a rating of values of words selected by a 20-item inventory to describe the pain rating index of sensation (PRIS) as well as affective nature of pain (PRIA) and evaluative measurement of pain (PRIE).

The number of words chosen (NWC) from the same category of 20 words is also recorded. This method is quite reliable.[47,117,282,386]

6. The regional analog scale is done by a 10-cm line drawn on a piece of paper. On an extreme of the line, the pain is indicated by a 0, and on the other extreme of the line the pain is indicated by 100. The patient then will apply an "x" mark where the patient considers the intensity and severity of the pain. This test also has been quite reliable.[157]

7. Localization of pain. The patient is asked to localize and draw the area of the pain on a preprinted human drawing. This is a good control in case of malingering or hysterical type of pain when the area the patient specifies does not necessarily correlate with the area that the examiner can elicit the pain.

BONE SCAN

The second diagnostic method of RSD is technetium bone scanning.[56,77,111,143,159,174–178,201] This is mainly helpful in the second and third stages and rarely in the first stage. It shows asymmetry of technetium uptake in the bones in the extremity involved with RSD. However, in the early stages, it usually points to the wrong side. For example, the patient may have RSD involving the right ankle and right knee, and yet the normal side may show an increased uptake of isotope rather than the abnormal side. In addition, this test is nonspecific, and many other conditions such as arthritis, infection, malignancy, and gout, can show the same abnormality.[110,174–176]

Since 1977, Kozin et al.[177] have shown the usefulness of scintigraphic radioisotope bone scanning in the diagnosis of RSD. The bone scanning quite frequently shows bilateral abnormalities[178] and in this regard points to the common phenomenon of RSD involving both extremities rather than one extremity.[178]

The confusing results of bone scan in different stages of RSD have been reported by Kozin.[175–178] Recently Block[511] has compared the different stages of RSD with the bone scan results. The Technetium-99 scintigraphy showed an increased blood flow in the involved joint in stage 1, but in stages 2 and 3 it showed a decreased blood flow in the same involved joint. Not infrequently, the report is pointing to an increased area of uptake of the Technetium. This is quite confusing to the clinician who realizes that the contralateral extremity is the one that is symptomatic and is causing problems for the patient.

After thermography, the radioisotope bone scanning is the most sensitive test in the diagnosis of RSD. As the RSD becomes chronic, the bilateral nature of the disease becomes more obvious on radioisotope bone scanning.

The bone scanning has a tendency for being positive either on the same side, opposite side, or on both sides of the vasoconstriction in the involved extremity causes a false positive scanning on the opposite extremity. In the later stages, the RSD is manifested on bone scanning with involvement of both extremities. In stages 3 and 4, the involved side shows more abnormality than the other side. As a result, there is tendency for confusion in the clinical correlation of bone scanning with the thermography. Other conditions such as infection may cause similar results.

In our series of 128 patients, the bone scan test has been diagnostic in 68 (53%) of RSD patients.

QSART SWEAT RESPONSE TEST

Low et al.[557,558] have utilized the quantative sweat response test (QSART) and thermoregularity sweat tests with as high as 80% abnormalities noted in small-fibroneuropathy patients. We have found these tests to be abnormal in RSD patients as well.[559]

SCR

Skin conductance response (SCR) is used in some laboratories based on the fact that disturbance of sympathetic dysfunction causes a disturbance of SCR. This is useful in assessment of effectiveness of sympathectomy postoperatively. It is not a sensitive test in the early stages of the illness.

CBV AND LDF

Measurement of capillary blood velocity (CBV) of the skin of the third or fourth fingers with a Leitz epi-illumination microscope combined with laser doppler flux (LDF) measurement[96,261,372] is quite sensitive in assessment of skin blood flow. The test shows an increase in skin and regional blood flow in early types of RSD. In more advanced stages the same areas show a reduction of blood flow. Between the acute and chronic stages, a steady-state stage occurs that is identical to normal skin blood flow (Table 17).

This test[96,261,372] is very sensitive, but can yield confusing results. The confusion is not necessarily due to temporal factors, but to the fact that advanced ephaptic RSD can cause a persistent increase in skin flow over the damaged area surrounded by decreased flow in adjacent areas.

NOREPINEPHRINE SPILLOVER

Meredith et al.[222] and Esler et al. measured the total and organ-specific norepinephrine in normal and in heart attack patients. They have noted that "in some patients major arrhythmias are associated with and caused by sustained and selective sympathetic dysfunction."

TABLE 17
Bilateral Stress Tests for Sympathetic Function in
Extremities: Schwartzman Method[19,22a]

30 seconds hyperventilation
Valsalva maneuver
Dynamometer static grip
Exercise
30 seconds immersion of hands or feet in 0°C water
  Laser doppler fluxmetry
  (Bonner and Tukey methods)

a Sympathetic stimulation: Schwartzman has outlined five methods of
   autonomic stimulation.[19,22] This measurement of sympathetic response usually shows bilateral changes pointing to a central origin
   of RSD.[19,22] As is the case with bone scan[176] and thermography, the
   doppler fluxmetry test is confusing because of the bilateral nature of
   RSD.

OTHER METHODS

Before discussing thermography, it should be mentioned that there are other methods that
are not as accurate or practical.

1. Starch test: checks the pattern of sweating — obviously too limited for measurement of
    sympathetic function.
2. Mercury-in-rubber strain gauge plethysmography: measures volume and circumference
    of the limb: not a specific or informative test for RSD.
3. Internal calorimetry: a needle calorimeter inserted in deep structures of an organ reads
    the temperature and indirectly measures blood flow. This traumatic test has no place in
    diagnosis of RSD.

USE OF THERMOGRAPHY IN RSD

"The biggest cause of trouble in the world today is that the stupid people are so sure about things, and the intelligent folks are so full of doubts."

Bertrand Russell

Diagnosing RSD without thermography is equivalent to diagnosing a heart attack without EKG. Of all the tests applied for the diagnosis of RSD, thermography is the most sensitive.[97,178,242] In early stages, thermography may show confusing results (Figures 4–6).

Infrared telethermography (Figures 2 and 3) is the most sensitive test in the diagnosis of RSD. It is not an accurate test for other causes of pain such as disc herniation or somatic nerve root dysfunction. Because it addresses itself purely to temperature differences and subtle temperature changes in different parts of the skin, and because it is quite sensitive and consistent, it provides a sensitive and accurate detail of the temperature pattern of the skin and it is the most practical and accurate test for early diagnosis of RSD.

Prior to the advent of thermography, the incidence of RSD among the chronic pain patients was approximately four times lower than after the advent of this test (Table 18). Whereas MRI and CAT scan as anatomical tests are most sensitive in diagnosing disc herniation, they are helpful in only $1/4$ of the chronic back pain problems. The EMG identifies the motor nerve dysfunction and the SSEP is most accurate for the diagnosis of sensory nerve dysfunction. The thermography should not be compared to these tests because it purely and exclusively addresses itself to the identification of thermatones. For example, in the case of electrical injuries, the damage to the upper extremity causes damage of the thermatones all the way up to the precordial region T2-T5 level. This is identified only with the help of thermography (see Electrical Injuries).

TABLE 18
Incidence of RSD

Prethermography	
Literature	1 to 2.5%
Our series of over 400 patients	5.7%
Postthermography	
Ecker, A: Thermology, 1985	21.5%
Our series of 482 patients: 101	22.0%

Thermography is an objective test[312] and has been shown to be equal to and at times better than other imaging test.[104,161,382,410,415] The inter-examiner agreement between single blind studies of different positions interpreting thermography has a consistency of over 80%.[50,59,410]

Thermography is done by measurement of natural infrared emission of human body heat with the help of infrared sensitive camera. A second, less commonly used method, contact thermography, measures minute temperature changes of the skin. Cholesterol crystals exposed to minor temperature changes undergo a change of polarity and color.

Thermography can detect 0.5–1°C temperature changes, but it evaluates only the 6-mm thickness of skin. It does not show the temperature changes deeper than 6 mm (muscle and bone temperature changes). However, the deeper structure injuries reflexly cause superficial skin temperature changes that can be measured by thermography.[428]

The main contribution of thermography to medicine has been its usefulness in early diagnosis of RSD. Obviously, in the third stage (RSA) that results in multiple pathologic fractures in the osteoporotic bone, the condition is far more resistant to therapy than RSD 1, which does not cause any significant bone pathology.

The late diagnosis in Wang's[398] group resulted in 55% success, and in our late diagnosis group it resulted in only 46% success. This is in contrast to a 77% success rate in early diagnosis in our group of patients. In ephaptic RSD (painful neuropathy) in Wang's group the success rate was 53% of the cases. In our ephaptic group the success rate was 48%.*

It becomes obvious that early diagnosis of RSD with the help of thermography — definitely earlier than 3 months after trauma — is quite essential in the successful management of such patients.

Early diagnosis is the single most important factor in determining the outcome of treatment of RSD.[227,269,308] Poplawski et al.[280] in reporting the results of treatment of RSD stated: "The most important factor in predicting improvement with treatment was a short interval (less than 6 months) between the onset of dystrophy and the administration of therapy."[280] Advanced forms of RSD are easy to diagnose but very hard to treat.

It is obvious that thermography is one of the most accurate diagnostic tools in the diagnosis of RSD. The only problem with the application of thermography in RSD is its hypersensitivity. In this regard, it is no different than CT or MRI (Table 16). The hypersensitivity along with deviation of sympathetic thermatomes from somatic dermatomes cause inaccuracies in application of thermography in nerve root injuries[130] (Figures 4a–c).

This hypersensitivity may cause a tendency for overinterpretation of thermography in RSD. Usually it is recommended that there be at least a 1°C temperature differential before an RSD is diagnosed.

This is quite a hypersensitive temperature differential, and may result in overinterpretation. It is best to limit the interpretation of RSD to 1.5–2°C, and ideally 2°C for the borderline cases.

Uematsu and his colleagues[379–382] applied thermography in the evaluation of 803 chronic pain patients. The abnormal thermographies were divided into nerve root dysfunction versus RSD. They found 42 RSD patients of whom 67% had more than a 2°C temperature drop on the painful side.

As is quite obvious, EMG was not useful in the diagnosis of RSD in these patients.

The other pitfall in the application of thermography in RSD is equating abnormal thermography with quantitative measurement of pain.

Thermography does have false positive results in patients who have had old injuries to their sympathetic nerve to the skin with no clinical pain being present.

The false positive results is a problem with all modern high-technology tests — be it thermography, CT, or MRI.

The MRI has contributed to excessive numbers of unnecessary disc surgeries by virtue of the fact that many ladies who have delivered a baby have a tendency to have an asymptomatic bulging of the L5-S1 disc.

A large number of patients with old cerebral dysfunctions, who are otherwise normal, are misdiagnosed as multiple sclerosis due to multiple innocent lesions in the brain on MRI that have no relationship to the patient's symptomatology (Table 16).

No specific test identifies the disease better than another test. The fancy tests tell us where the lesion is. A careful history tells us what disease we are dealing with. No test identifies "pain" better than another test.

Thermography, by virtue of identifying thermatomal abnormalities in peripheral nerves, may be helpful in the diagnosis of nerve root dysfunction.[93] However, this is no one-to-one relationship.[272]

---

* Morphine pump treatment was not included in the studies due to short period of follow-up. Morphine pump seems to provide over 95% success.

OBJECTIVE VS. SUBJECTIVE PAIN

Contrary to general belief, pain is not a "purely subjective" symptom. The presence of pain as the patient complains can be objectively corroborated.

If a patient is undergoing an acute myocardial infarct and complains of pain in the jaw or neck or chest, usually the patient also has overt manifestations of severe pain. These consist of grayish discoloration of skin, excessive sweating secondary to sympathetic hyperactivity, blood pressure changes, and pulse changes.

However, all of the pains and especially chronic pain are not this obvious. Yet, with the help of neurophysiological tests, one can corroborate the presence of pain as the source of an organic assault to the body.

Such tests may measure the sensory, autonomic, or motor function of the area involved: SSEP is specific for sensory, thermography for autonomic nerve fibers, and EMG for motor nerve fibers.

Traditionally the clinician has a tendency to try to find the cause of pain by anatomical tests such as X-ray, CT scan, myelography, or MRI. The anatomical tests are usually more misleading and are accompanied by a higher number of false positive results or false negative results than neurophysiological tests.

A patient who is complaining of chest pains does not and should not undergo MRI of the chest to find out the cause of the chest pain. In this situation, a simple two-century-old physiological test, the EKG, easily helps establish a diagnosis of the pain.

However, for some unknown reason, the same simple principle has not been applied for other neurologic types of pain.

The patient may have emotional neck pain or back pain, and yet MRI may show bulging of the discs in the spine. That becomes an excuse for the surgeon to operate on the bulging disc, which usually has no relationship to the original cause of the pain. As a result, the surgery becomes a new source of pain for the patient. The reverse is true with regard to the fact that usually surgeons or neurologists order MRIs for patients with neck and back pain; if the MRI is negative, they refer the patient to a psychiatrist. The experience of pain clinics (Rosomoff[306]) as well as our experience confirms that only one quarter to one third of the patients with neck and back pain suffer from disc herniation; the rest have other causes (Table 7).

The surgeon may go one step further and order neurophysiological tests such as EMG for the diagnosis of the source of pain. EMG mainly studies the motor function of the nerves and limited sensory nerve conduction times. This test cannot diagnose the cause of an autonomic type of pain such as RSD or pain due to partial sensory nerve root dysfunction.[306]

Sensory nerve root dysfunction is better evaluated by evoked potential tests,[93,391] motor function by EMG test, and autonomic function by thermography.[73]

RELIABILITY OF THERMOGRAPHY

Thermography, which is a direct measurement of the temperature controlled by the sympathetic nervous system, is most reliable for evaluation of RSD.[575] The normal human values have been standardized, replicated, and proven valid and reproducible.[577,578]

By the same token, it does not have a one-to-one correlation with motor or sensory nerve root distribution of pain. Even though thermography can be quite informative in the evaluation of low back pain syndrome patients,[59,305] it does not necessarily identify a specific nerve root as the cause of pain.[576] This is due to the fact that thermatomes and dermatomes do not necessarily sumperimpose each other in an exact fashion (Figure 4a).

Thermography is quite an objective test,[312] which is much more sensitive than simple observation of the patient or tactile examination of the patient or a bone scan measurement for the diagnosis of RSD. **At the present time, no other test is as sensitive as thermography for RSD.**[575] Obviously, thermography is not as accurate to identify dermatomal pathology.[381,576] In turn, **EMG, MRI,** and **SSEP** are incapable of diagnosing RSD.

Unless a carefully controlled technique is used, thermography, like any other test, is apt to show too much artifact, false positive, and false negative results. These standards have been well established by Wexler and Chafetz[410] in 1987, and the standard position has been outlined by the academy of neuormuscular thermography in 1989.[352]

With proper technique, thermography has been demonstrated to be equal to or at times better than other imaging tests.[104,161,382,410,415]

Thermography measures a physiological function of the body, and although from day to day the physiological status of the body may change, the symmetry vs. asymmetry of the thermographic pattern on the two sides of the body stays quite consistent. The normal control symmetry vs. the abnormal asymmetrical patterns have stayed consistent from day to day. However, the abnormality may improve or deteriorate, which may make the asymmetry more prominent or less prominent.[380,408] The consistency and interexaminer agreement between single-blind studies of different interpreters of thermography have shown a consistency of 80 to 100%.[50,59,410]

Thermography is a useful test as long as it is performed properly. Comparing thermography with CT scanning in patients with low back pain and sciatica, an 84% and higher accuracy has been reported.[99,272] Similar high rates of correlation have been reported comparing thermography and surgical findings. A comparison of thermography with EMG, myelography, and SSEP, shows similar high correlations.[99,272] Thermography's main use and the most valuable contribuion is the early diagnosis of RSD.

11

Prevention of RSD

"The most important factor in predicting improvement ... was less than 6 months between onset of RSD and the administration of
therapy."

Poplawski et al.[280]

OUTLINE OF PREVENTION

I.   Early diagnosis (thermography, bone scan)
      The magic word is diagnosis and treatment before 6 months
II.   Early physiotherapy
      Avoid ice application
      Avoid braces
      Avoid immobilization
      Avoid alcohol
      Avoid litigation
      Avoid narcotics, barbiturates, BZs, (e.g., Fiorinal, Fioricet, Valium, Halcion, etc.)
III. Avoid surgery
      A. Especially cutting around the scars on the dorsum of the foot
      B. Unnecessary surgery for nerve roots contusion misdiagnosed as
              Tardy ulnar palsy
              Disc herniation
      C. Unnecessary arthroscopy
      D. Amputation (for Sudek's atrophy and fractures)
      E. Sympathectomy
      F. RSD involving foot is misdiagnosed by some podiatrists as "neuroma"; surgery on
          the foot results in intractable RSD
IV.   Not applying preventive measures results in acceleration of Stages I through III; by
      stage IV, the patient's life is in danger of suicide or heart attack

In no disease, short of some rare fatal infectious diseases, is prevention as important as in
treatment of reflex dystrophy dysfunction.
    Prevention is important in prevention of the trauma, and even more important in prevention
of the more severe stages of the disease.

The more aggressively the illness is treated in the first stage (reflex sympathetic temporary dysfunction, RSDF), the better the chances are to prevent the development of the second stage (reflex sympathetic dystrophy, RSD).

It is even more important to prevent the development of the third stage (reflex sympathetic atrophy, RSA) because this is the stage where the rate of success drops drastically, and this is the stage where the patient is at the risk of ending up with unnecessary operations such as amputation and sympathectomy.

PREVENTIVE MEASURES

The following principles play a major role in prevention of RSD and its further deterioration:

1. Early diagnosis, especially with the help of thermography.
2. Early aggressive physical therapy.
3. Avoidance of the unnecessary use of braces, crutches, casts, and immobilization when the patient has a soft tissue injury rather than a fracture or major ligament tear.
4. Avoidance of the use of ice on the involved area. Ice is the treatment of choice for acute somatic pain. It is also instigator, aggravator, and perpetuator of RSD because of its vasoconstrictive effect.
5. Avoidance of alcohol in any amount.
6. Avoidance of narcotics and benzodiazepines in any amount and at any stage, except for clonopin used for seizure disorder.
7. Avoidance of unnecessary surgery such as cutting and suturing in the area of scars, unnecessary surgery such as done for back or cervicolumbar spinal pain when the patient's problem is only nerve root contusion or chronic pain, or when the MRI or myelography do not corroborate the exact abnormality or the EMG, somatosensory evoked response, or thermography. The same is true with unnecessary operations such as amputation and sympathectomy and injection with steroids to the area of ephaptic scar.

Arthroscopy should be avoided until absolutely necessary because the trauma of arthroscopy can cause injury to the sensory nerves around the knee and start ephaptic RSD.

Finally, unnecessary surgery for improperly diagnosed carpal tunnel syndrome, tardy ulnar palsy, or rotator cuff tear should be avoided.

EARLY DIAGNOSIS OF RSD

> "Sir, it is no matter what you teach them first, anymore than what leg you should put into your breeches first. Sir, you may stand disputing ... but in the meantime your breech is bare."
>
> Dr. Samuel Johnson, 1771

REFLEX SYMPATHETIC DYSFUNCTION

When RSD is diagnosed and treated in the first few weeks, the treatment is rewarded by a high rate of success and cure.

With the advent of thermography, there is no justification in allowing reflex sympathetic dysfunction to progress to the later stages when the condition can be diagnosed quite accurately early in the course of the illness.

Thermography is useless in identifying specific nerve root dysfunction because the thermatomes that are in the distribution of emphatic nerve roots are not accurately correspondent to the dermatomes that are representative of the pressure on the nerve roots in the spinal canal.

Thermography exclusively specifies dysfunction in the thermatome of the sympathetic nerves and is of limited use in diagnosing which level of the cervicolumbar spinal canal is the disc herniation causing the patient's problems.

Obviously, less than one-third of all chronic back and neck pains is due to cervical disc herniation.[306] Even then, there are much better tests such as EMG, MRI, or myelography to identify nerve root dysfunction.

Of the three different types of peripheral nerve dysfunction, the sensory nerve dysfunction is best studied by somatosensory evoked potentials (SEP) and to a lesser extent by sensory nerve conduction tests.

The autonomic nerve dysfunction is best studied by thermography and the motor peripheral nervous dysfunction is best studied by electromyography (EMG).

Only in the latter part of the second stage of reflex sympathetic dystrophy and especially in the third stage of reflex sympathetic atrophy can a bedside examination identify this illness with certainity. Otherwise thermography is the most accurate test for early diagnosis of reflex sympathetic dysfunction. The value of thermography is practically limited to diagnosis of RSD. It is far more accurate than bone scan, and it has less false positive results or confusing identification of the side of pathology than isotope bone scanning.

Table 6 demonstrates the results of thermography in ipsilateral and contralateral extremities in a temporal fashion in regard to RSD of disuse and ephaptic RSD. It is imperative to diagnose reflex sympathetic dysfunction as early as possible to prevent the development of Stages II and III.

Aggressive physiotherapy and application of nerve blocks are essential in the prevention of the deterioration of RSD. Also it is the only effective treatment for reflex sympathetic dysfunction secondary to RSD of disuse.

Physiotherapy prevents the development of the second and third stages of RSD. As a preventive and therapeutic modality physiotherapy plays even a more important role in RSD than in Parkinson's disease. In the latter illness, any treatment is apt to fail, and Parkinson's disease is apt to progressively deteriorate unless treatment is accompanied by aggressive physiotherapy. However, the consequences of lack of physiotherapy in RSD are even more serious than in Parkinson's disease.

Therapeutic modality should be adjusted according to the type of RSD. After the proper diagnosis is made with regard to RSD of disuse vs. ephaptic RSD, the therapeutic modalities of physiotherapy are quite different. Obviously, application of ice, TNS, or trigger point injection into the area of the scar has a serious consequence with rapid deterioration of RSD.

On the other hand, the same treatment applied to the referred pain point and trigger point away from the scar region can be quite helpful in treatment of ephaptic RSD.

Without the help of thermography, an accurate diagnosis of ephaptic RSD as differentiated from RSD of disuse is quite difficult, and the diagnosis can be made only after the disease has become too progressive for any successful treatment.

Avoidance of the use of braces and casts is quite essential in the prevention of the formation of RSD.

It is quite common for a patient who has upper extremity injuries to arrive at an emergency room and end up leaving with a sling around his neck. Although done with the good intention of the doctors and nurses in the emergency room, immobilization can have serious consequences, causing or aggravating RSD of disuse or ephaptic RSD. This kind of immobilization actively reduces the proprioceptive impulses to the spinal cord and leaves the anterolateral horn cells of the spinal cord uninhibited with secondary vasoconstriction and development of RSD.

Obviously a patient with a fracture should be given a cast and a patient with a major tear in the ligament of the joint should be given some form of immobilization, but it is safer for the ER physician to leave it up to the orthopedist to decide if the patient needs long-term immobilization.

Application of ice may be quite helpful in acute stages of RSD when it is given in the area of referred pain such as over the posterior cervical region in a patient with injury to the neck and shoulder; but if the patient has a scar causing RSD of disuse, application of ice in this area is only going to make the adjacent area of the scar become colder and is going to result in a significant temperature differential between the adjacent area of the scar and the warm area of acute region of the scar. This in turn causes more hyperpathic input of pain to the central nervous system with aggravation of RSD of disuse.

If there is any suspicion or suggestion that the patient is starting to have reflex sympathetic dysfunction, it should be treated with heat rather than ice.

AVOIDANCE OF ALCOHOL

Avoidance of alcohol is discussed in detail in Chapter 9 (Alcohol Abuse and RSD). The use of any volume of alcoholic beverages during the treatment for RSD is not only contraindicated but is tantamount to total failure of treatment.

Alcohol on a short-term basis within a few hours and in large doses is an analgesic. However, after a few hours, the withdrawal effect causes five problems:

1. Acid rain phenomenon (destruction of nerve cells in the brain stem, which are responsible for the formation of hormones and neurotransmitters).
2. Gate effect of alcohol (gate theory): the use of one addicting drug opens the gate (demand) for other similar addicting drugs, e.g., alcohol opens the gate to narcotics and tranquilizers (see Chapter 9, Alcohol Abuse and RSD).
3. Alcohol increases the hyperoxide activity in the area of damage to the soft tissue, which further aggravates the soft tissue pathology.
4. Alcohol causes dehydration of the soft tissues and aggravation of pain. This especially is the case in disc desiccation and early spondylosis formation in the spine of drinkers.
5. Alcohol reduces endorphins as well as sex hormones — especially estrogen — with secondary aggravation of pain and depression.

ACID RAIN

Acid rain term refers to the fact that alcohol causes death of nerve cells, and as a result, proportionately reduces the biogenic amines, neurotransmitters, and hormones secreted by the nerve cells — especially in the brain stem (Figures 21a and 21b).

The following discussion regarding the effect of alcohol refers specifically to the long-term effect of alcohol. Viewing the acute ingestion of alcohol, the effect may be temporarily opposite of what alcohol does to the CNS in the long term.

For example, during acute ingestion of 2 to 4 ounces of alcohol, the patient usually feels excited, uninhibited, and actually pain free. The intoxication of the frontal lobe nerve cells on an acute basis results in the patient feeling so free of pain and so careless that it imitates the use of stimulants such as cocaine, dexedrine, or Ritalin.

The patient may then become hypomanic and feel omnipotent. During this stage, the reduction of the inhibitory effect of the cerebral cortex causes rapid thinking and more creative function of the brain.

Writers use this stage of intoxication to create their masterpieces or to compose their poetry.

Businessmen use this stage of alcohol ingestion to sell their products or to give oratory lectures.

Teenagers use this stage of alcohol ingestion to feel more free to talk to the opposite sex and not be shy about it.

In this stage, the effects of alcohol on pain, the heart, and the autonomic nervous system are identical to cocaine stimulation. As a result, the patient develops tachycardia, hypertension, and hyperactivity of the autonomic nervous system.

As is the case with chronic pain manifesations, be it RSD or any other form of chronic pain, the deleterious effect of alcohol mostly is due to the long-term effect of alcohol on the central nervous system (see Chapter 9, Alcohol Abuse and RSD).

EFFECT OF ALCOHOL ON LIMBIC SYSTEM

The three structures — limbic system, hypothalamus, and brain stem — not only have a rich and two-way feedback interaction. In the case of the limbic system and brain stem, the two structures are practically identical and overlapping phylogenetically as well as chemically. The connections of the limibic system to the brain stem are so abundant that actually the brain stem should be considered as a part of the limbic system (Figures 12a, 21a, and 21b).

Functionally, the brain stem as a part of the limbic system, through its extensive electro-chemical modulatory effect on the central and peripheral nervous system, it is responsible for diurnal functions of the body. It controls the sleep/wakeful cycle, and controls the changes in mood and the rate of activity of the CNS as well as the endocrine system.

Through the hypothalamic brain stem axis, the CNS controls the daily fluctuation of hormones in the endocrine system and as a result influences the states of depression, agitation, tranquility, etc.

The brain stem wakes us up in the morning and puts us to sleep at night. During the day it provides neurotransmitters and hormones that control the daily response toward stress and toward the necessity of fight and flight.

The brain stem does all of this by having ascending and descending excitatory and inhibitory feedback systems that control every aspect of our daily activity from sleep/wakefulness to happiness/depression mood fluctuations to control of instinctual endocrine functions such as appetite, sex, rage, tranquility, or love or hatred type of instincts.

Histochemical studies of the brain stem[30,31,140,160,164,198,270,271,347,400] and cerebral hemisphere reveal the presence of neurotransmitters, ACTH, endorphins, 5-HTP, and substance P

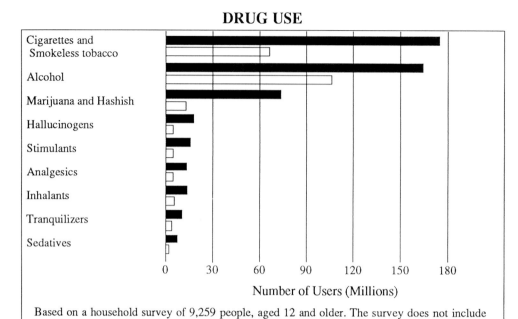

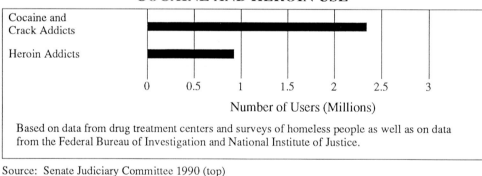

FIGURE 27. Incidence of drug addiction. Sources: Senate Judiciary Committee (1990), FBI, National Institute of Justice, and Centers for the homeless. (This figure is modified from p. 96 of *Scientific American*, March 1991.)

in unlimited number of nuclei in the brain stem such as raphe median, raphe nuclei, periaqueductal gray matter, and frontal lobes (Figures 12a, 21a, and 21b).

These areas are rich in neurotransmitters such as endorphins, which provide endogenous relief of pain, and cholecystokinin (CCK), which controls appetite and facilitates motor activity. There are many other biogenic amines such as ACTH that not only stimulate peripheral endocrine organs but also stimulate endorphin formation and play a major role in control of chronic pain.[40]

Substance P is rich in dorsal raphe nuclei and periaquaductal gray, and plays a major modulatory role in excitation and inhibition of pain through ascending and descending fibers to the thalamus and spinal cord.

Luteinizing hormone (LH) plays a major role in stimulation of the sex hormone, which is quite important both in combatting depression as well as providing relief of pain by enhancement of healing of soft tissues and counteracting dryness of soft tissues as well as counteracting osteoporosis (Table 24).

The list is quite long, and only some of these neurotransmitters are recognized.[160]

The above-mentioned gray matter in the brain stem in the medical literature of the 1960s and 1970s has been referred to under the terminology "reticular activating system". However, this reticular system is putative. It is not only activating, but is an inactivating, excitatory, and inhibitory modulator of all the diurnal functions, e.g., wakefulness, sleep, endocrine function, and control of mood and pain.

Alcohol destroys this entire system by killing the nerve cells that generate such important neurotransmitters and hormones.

Cocaine stimulates the dopaminergic function of this system at the expense of not allowing the reticular system to provide serotonin and other neurotransmitters.

The use of external benzodiazepines (BZ) depletes the system of its own endo BZ and causes withdrawal in the form of panic, insomnia, phobia, and severe anxiety.

Narcotics inhibit the formation of endorphins (enkephalin and met-enkephalin). The endorphin depletion of the system results in phobia, panic, severe pain, headaches, insomnia, and a feeling of alarm and impending death.

RSD AND THE EFFECT OF DRUGS ON THE BRAIN STEM

As outlined above, the sedative drugs such as alcohol, narcotics, benzodiazepines, and barbiturates obviously paralyze the natural modulation and formation of similar chemicals in the brain stem with resultant pain, anxiety, and depression, which are the salient features of RSD. Consequently, the disease develops with more rapid progression and deterioration.

Other drugs, which are socially classified as "foods", should be avoided, and the drugs that are called foods have the same deleterious effect on RSD as small amounts of alcohol, cocaine, dexedrine, or Ritalin have on this illness. These unnatural foods aggravate the RSD not only in the extremities, but also in the craniocervical region. The aggravation of RSD in the craniocervical region is traditionally classified as migraine headache, and avoidance of these artificial junk foods does benefit the patients who suffer from migraine headaches, RSD, or attention deficit.

AVOIDANCE OF LITIGATION

Litigation delays proper diagnosis and treatment, and the delay exponentially increases the failure rate of treatment. Of the 12 patients in our series who eventually required Morphine pump treatment because all else failed, the treatment was delayed by an average of 37 months. Nine of the 12 patients were in litigation due to Workers' Compensation injuries.

Any kind of emotional distress is apt to perpetuate and deteriorate any chronic pain, especially RSD.

Legal settlement and avoidance of prolonged litigation are quite helpful in management of this illness.

The following case is a prototype of a common work injury resulting in chronic pain and RSD with disastrous results.

Our macabre story starts with a happily married 24-year-old gentleman who works at the local department store. He accidentally slips on a wet spot on the floor. Caught off guard, he has quite a fall with injuries to his back and his left foot, which is caught under the weight of his body. He develops severe back pain and left foot pain. His true diagnosis is injury to the sensory nerve fibers of the ankle on the left side with secondary RSD aggravated by inactivity as well as bruises to the bones and joints in the back. These usually are of a temporary nature.

He reports his accident to his boss. It is considered workers' compensation, and his company sends him to an "insurance company doctor". The patient discusses the entire case with his lawyer who advises him to see a "plaintiff doctor". Under the direction and advice of the two adversaries, he goes to both doctors. The first one diagnoses a mild sprain with no disability and instructs the patient to return to work immediately. The second doctor diagnoses the patient as suffering from severe injuries to the sciatic nerve, the lumbosacral region, and nerves of the left foot, and immobilizes the injured limb. He gives the patient a cane to use. Inactivity, guarding the extremity, and peripheral sensory nerve damage cause cold extremity and RSD.

Two weeks after the accident he has followed the advice of his family physician — spending his days in bed and taking isocodone and diazepam for pain. Inactivity is perpetuating the pain. Due to reduction in cerebral endorphins and endoBZ's the patient wakes up every 3 hours so he can take more medication.

The confusion in diagnosis and the conflict in his treatment plans cause the patient to become depressed, distrustful, and severely concerned about his future. The isocodone and diazepam aggravate the depression. His job is in danger because he has not shown up for work as recommended by the first doctor.

To solve the conflict of the two diagnoses and the opposing treatments, he goes to a surgeon. The surgeon obtains an MRI. The MRI shows some red herring type abnormality in his back (bulging disc) which has no relationship with the patient's pain. On the basis of MRI, the surgeon operates on the patient. Three months after the accident, the patient has two causes of pain: the original pain that has become chronic, and the new pain due to trauma of surgery. More isocodone, more diazepam, more depression, and more inactivity follow.

Eventually after a year of misery, at last he is forced to go back to work. At work, due to insomnia secondary to chronic pain, and addicting medications, he sustains a second minor injury and loses his job. Another surgeon opines that the patient needs a lumbar fusion. The fusion is done. The result is obvious: failed back. By now, not only the patient's back has failed, but he has been so depressed, irritable, impotent, and in so much financial trouble that he loses his wife. He finds relief in alcohol and narcotics. He tries to commit suicide unsuccessfully, and becomes another victim of the miracle of modern medicine.

The chronic pain by and large gradually disappears unless the following factors perpetuate and make it persistent. The following factors are called the five D's of chronic pain. These consist of dependence, dysfunction, disability, drug abuse, and dramatization.

1.   Dependence: the patient may passively or aggressively need the pain to deal with his job and family problems.
2.   Dysfunction is the second factor in perpetuating the pain, especially the pain of RSD. This is due to inactivity. Advising the patient to stay in bed is usually the worst thing to do for the chronic pain patient. This makes the patient more susceptible to stress and perpetuates the pain. This results in RSD, obesity, aggravation of depression, and dysfunction of the endocrine system with less desire for exercise or sex.
3.   Disability rating is the third most important factor in perpetuation of pain. Without the disability rating, the patient is liable to lose any refund for his disability.
4.   Drug abuse. At present, the most common cause of perpetuation and aggravation of chronic pain is the unnecessary and vicarious use of narcotics. Unfortunately, for too long the attitude toward chronic pain has been either to "cut it out or cover it up" with narcotics. Neither of these two (surgery or narcotics) has any place in the treatment of chronic pain. The use of narcotics stops the brain from making its own endorphins. As a result, every 3 to 4 hours the body becomes totally dependent on narcotics.
    The liberal attitude of physicians toward ethanol intake aggravates the chronic pain.

5.   Dramatization is an important factor in chronic pain, resulting in unnecessary surgery, unnecessary hospitalization, unnecessary tests, treatment, and a vicious circle of chronic pain-surgery-acute pain-chronic pain-surgery.

The impressive role of a family member in perpetuation of pain is a spouse who keeps looking for an "organic cause" for the pain. He takes his wife from doctor to doctor to prove that it is not in her head. The family may be supportive, with ameleorating effect on chronic pain, or may be manipulative with aggravating effect on chronic pain.

The following are some fallacies about chronic pain:

1.   "It's all in your head." Obviously every pain is felt not in the "fingers" but in the head.
2.   If there is nothing that needs an operation, then it is "psychosomatic". The psychosomatic terminology is archaic, nonscientific, and remnant of old Freudian days. As far as pain is concerned, there is no difference between psyche and soma. A gangrene of the right big toe is just as disturbing to the psyche as the painful loss of a child. As a matter of fact, serious psychotic illnesses are not accompanied by pain, and psychotics rarely complain of pain. What is called psychosomatic is a terminology to cover the diagnostic shortfall. With the help of PET and brain mapping, the development of frontal lobe dysfunction has been demonstrated in chronic pain (Figure 26.)
3.   Bedrest as treatment for pain. Bedrest and inactivity are distressful and aggravate the chronic pain.
4.   Pain medication for treatment of chronic pain. Pain medication of choice for RSD and other forms of chronic pain is antidepressants — not narcotics.
5.   "If you don't need an operation, then your pain is not real." Rare cases are helped with operation for the chronic pain.
6.   Acupuncture, as a cure for chronic pain, is nothing but a charlatan approach and is absolutely useless. In controlled trials of treatment of chronic pain, acupuncture has had the same success as placebo treatment. It is properly used in China as an anesthetic because of the fact that this treatment blocks pain acutely and the surgeon can operate under the effect of acupuncture. However, the effect of acupuncture wears off in a matter of several minutes. By the time the chronic pain patient has left the acupuncturist's office, the effect wears off as well. So it is no treatment or cure, but is a waste of time and money for the patient.

12

Management of RSD

"What physic, what chirurgery, what wealth,
favor, authority can relieve, bear out, assuage,
or expel a troubled conscience? A quiet mind
cureth all."

Richard Burton, 1622

SUMMARY OF MANAGEMENT

1. No surgery
2. Early diagnosis — ideally in first 2–3 months (early thermography when indicated)
3. Early physiotherapy, early mobilization
4. Early nerve block (earlier than first 6 months), repetitive blocks as needed
5. Throw away crutches and other assistive devices
6. Detoxify early: discontinue alcohol, cigarettes, benzodiazepines, and narcotics
7. No systemic corticosteroids
8. Limit the use of corticosteroids to epidural blocks, regional blocks, articular facet injections, and trigger point injections
9. ACTH helps chronic pain treatment (it is not a corticosteroid)
10. Antidepressants are analgesics of choice for chronic pain in all its forms including RSD; avoid tricyclics that cause hypotension and poor erection
11. Management of insomnia; avoid benzodiazepines
12. Team work essential: physiatrist, anesthesiologist, and a neurologist with training background in neuroendocrinology and neuropharmacology
13. If all fails, in advanced cases, Morphine pump provides good relief.

EARLY DIAGNOSIS

The physicians are trained to suspect RSD only after it becomes clinically obvious (stages 3 and 4). Again, the diagnosis is indisputible, but the treatment is met with almost certain failure.

RSD is very easily and successfully treated in stage one and two, but is very difficult to diagnose at stages one and two. The reverse is true for stages three and four which are easy to diagnose and very difficult to treat.

Early diagnosis is the most important factor in determining the outcome of treatment.[227,269,308] After diagnosis is made, aggressive multidisciplinary treatment is essential.

TABLE 19
Do's and Don't's in Management of RSD

Do's: Aggressive management
- Early diagnosis
- Physiotherapy and hydrotherapy
- Throw away assistive devices, i.e., cane crutches, wheelchair, cast, walker, brace
- Start weight-bearing: even in osteoporotic fractures of small bones of the foot
- Trigger point injections; articular facet nerve blocks and injection
- Chemical block: procardia, calcium blockers, Catapres
- Sympathetic ganglion block or regional block
- Noninvasive TNS
- Correction of diet
- Stop narcotics, alcohol, and smoking
- Antidepressants
- ACTH instead of corticosteroids
- Limit the use of corticosteroids to
    Trigger point injection
    Epidural injection
    Regional block
- If all the above fail, use a morphine pump

Don'ts: Avoid the following
- Temptation of surgery
- Assistive devices
- Application of ice
- Sympathectomy
- Amputation
- Invasive stimulants, i.e., spinal cord and cerebral implants
- Rhizotomy, cingulotomy, and tractotomy
- Treatment with barbiturates or receptor-site binding benzodiazepines (clonazepam and oxazepam are the least binding)
- Sleeping pills with the exception of chloral hydrate and trazodone (increases REM)

RSD is best managed by a multidisciplinary therapeutic team approach.[131] As a form of chronic pain, simple drug treatment or surgery are apt to fail. Not only does sympathectomy show no significant long-term benefit, but other invasive treatments such as cingulomotomy,[313] thalamotomy, and depth electrode stimulation are doomed to fail in the long run. The use of pulse-generating stimulators such as epidural stimulation is usually effective in the first 9 to 18 months. Afterward, the CNS ignores the persistent digital (timelocked) stimulation. Alternately, multidisciplinary treatment is quite beneficial in RSD patients.[85,100,122,166,173,182,209,294,426]

In RSD of disuse, it is not unusual to cure the patient in early stages with physiotherapy, TNS, and proper medications without any need for sympathetic block.[199,364,421]

Assistive devices such as cane, crutches, brace, and cast should be discontinued. Weight-bearing, even in spite of osteoporosis of small bones of the foot, is essential and prevents the need for amputation.

PHYSIOTHERAPY

> "I believe that anyone can conquer fear by
> doing things he fears to do, provided he keeps
> doing them until he gets a record of success-
> ful experiences behind him."
>
> Mrs. Eleanor Roosevelt

The number one key to success in treatment of all forms of RSD[199,298,308] is physiotherapy. The sooner it is applied, the better the results. This form of treatment increases proprioception to the spinal cord, resulting in inhibition of an overactive sympathetic system. It also increases circulation to the extremity with secondary central inhibition of the sympathetic nervous system.

It counteracts immobilization of the joints and formation of trigger points and calcium deposits (bursitis). It prevents shoulder-hand syndrome and other forms of pain in the extremity secondary to RSD. It stimulates the formation of endorphins, and, as a result, relieves the pain. In addition, passive exercises as well as TNS help the development of Melzack's phenomenon of the stimulation of A fibers, which inhibit the C fiber input of pain at the spinal cord level.

Physiotherapy should not be limited to 2 or 3 days a week in the physiotherapy department. It should be continued at home several times a day.

The physiotherapist should mainly serve as instructor and counselor to help the patient overcome the fear of activity.

The physiotherapist should emphasize the importance of physiotherapy during all waking hours rather than just 2 or 3 days a week in the physical therapy department.

Application of moist heat (with thermophore hydroculator), massage with a dry towel, and traction (head-of-bed, as well as pelvic traction) should not be limited to two or three times a week, but should be done on a daily basis even after the patient returns to work.

The patient's relatives play a major role in regard to achievement of proper physiotherapy. A caring loved one, be it a spouse, friend, or parent, can make a big difference. Application of massage, helping the patient with application of traction, and encouraging the patient to become active and move around are important roles played by the relatives.

The patient should be instructed that without increase in activity and without exercise, there is no hope for successful treatment.

If there is **legal entanglement** regarding the nature of trauma, the sooner the case is settled, the better off the patient is; and the sooner the patient is instructed to return to work, the better the outcome of treatment.

Early application of physiotherapy as well as occupational therapy can make a big difference in the outcome of treatment.

MASSAGE

The application of massage is both preventive and curative in the management of trigger point.

Massage as well as traction should not be applied only at the physiotherapy department two or three times a week. The patient should be supplied with instruction in the use of the above-mentioned two modalities. These treatments should occur two or three times a day.

The massage can be done with a dry towel: the patient applies the towel to the posterior cervical region and the hands are used in a see-saw motion. This provides good massage, generates heat, and mechanically disseminates the trigger point to adjacent tissues. In turn, the increased circulation absorbs the chemicals accumulated at the trigger point.

AVOID ICE PACK APPLICATION

The sympathetic system is stimulated by cold. This stimulation results in aggravation and exaggeration of RSD. Moist heat does the opposite.

Whereas ice pack is the treatment of choice for acute soft tissue injuries, it is contraindicated in the complex chronic pain of RSD. If an ice pack helps the patient, then RSD is not the cause of the pain.

TRACTION

In patients suffering from RSD due to nerve root injuries, traction is an effective mode of therapy. Gentle traction relaxes the paraspinal muscles, provides proper proprioception, and counteracts aggravation of RSD. It widens the intervertebral foramina and relieves pressure on the nerve roots secondary to paraspinal spasm.

Traction with small weights such as 6 to 7 pounds for cervical spine and 15 to 20 pounds for the pelvic region is quite effective in prevention of formation of trigger point as well as prevention of muscle spasm, and formation of pain chemicals.

Proper instruction is quite essential for success of traction. If the axis of the rope of cervical traction is not continuous with the axis of the cervical spine, the patient may develop occipital neuralgia or painful TMJ complication.

Simultaneous head-of-bed and pelvic **traction** application on at least a daily or two to three times a day basis is quite helpful in treatment of cervical sprain and lumbar sprain and prevention of chronic neck and back pain.

It is obvious that with such small weight applied, as mentioned above, the goal is not to correct a dislocation or a disc herniation, but to achieve relief of pain and muscle spasm as well as **generating proper proprioception in the muscles of the neck and back**, hence, effectively counteracting RSD.

HYDROTHERAPY

The most effective form of hydrotherapy is soaking in **ocean water**, which has seven times the osmolality of blood. It dialyzes the algogenic substances through the skin. The second, more practical form, is soaking the extremity in epsom salt and hot water two to three times a day. Third, swimming is an effective physiotherapy.

Hydrotherapy plays a major role in helping the patient with physiotherapy mobilization as well as removal of rogue oxygen, substance P, and other painful chemicals at the trigger point area and at the area of nerve damage.

DISCONTINUATION OF ASSISTIVE DEVICES

As long as the patient is using canes, crutches, or a wheelchair, there is no hope for correction of RSD.

In advanced stages of diabetic neuropathy, Sudek's osteoporosis and pathologic fractures rapidly destroy the small bones of the foot. In such patients, weight-bearing corrects the hyperemia and osteoporosis with resultant healing of the fractures. Weight-bearing is not difficult in these patients because the bones are painless secondary to diabetic neuropathy.

In four such patients, weight-bearing on the fractured foot prevented the need for amputation.

Amputation in these patients has a disastrous result. The amputation is above the level of pathology where the nociceptive nerves are relatively intact and become the source of severe stump neuralgia and phantom pain.

It is a common practice among emergency room physicians, hand surgeons, and hand therapists to use a wrist brace or elbow brace to immobilize the hand or elbow. This immobilization is a major contributor to RSD of disuse and immobilizing the extensor and supinator muscles with resultant hyperactivity of the flexor and pronator muscles. As a result, when the braces are discontinued, the RSD extremity stays in a pronated and flexd positions. It will take repeated sympathetic blocks and extensive physiotherapy to correct such iatrogenic complications.

TRIGGER POINT INJECTION

Trigger point (Figure 22) is a "a focus of hyperirritability in muscle or fascia that can cause pain".[340]

Trigger point injection (TPI) is the treatment of choice for problems of referred pain secondary to inactivity and other causes of RSD.

"Myofascial" source of pain is a painful focus, which quite commonly is a source of referred pain with few exceptions. It is usually a cold area on thermography. It should not be mistaken for the area of scar, which is the source of ephaptic RSD and is hot on thermography, but it can be very close to or quite a distance away from the scar (see Chapter 8).

The trigger point usually is a referred pain quite a distance away from the point of origination of the pain. It is different from injury to the ligaments around a joint, calcium formation around the tendons due to inactivity, or a partial tear in the nerve or muscles underlying the skin.

Myofascial trigger points are not limited to RSD patients and can be present in many forms of musculoskeletal and bone and joint diseases. However, the **trigger points are quite common in RSD patients**.[138,227,269,308]

For management of trigger points, it is quite essential to determine the nature of the pathology of the trigger point; this makes the treatment easier. For example, if the trigger point is referred pain or pain due to disturbance of function of the posterior rami of the nerve roots, traction would be quite effective.

Trigger point injection, especially in the form of **spinal articular facet** injection, is very helpful in taking away the pain and enabling the patient to mobilize the extremity. Usually one or two injections are enough, but at times the patient may need repeated injections. The injections are not dose related, and even small doses of chemicals such as Depo-Medrol® are quite effective in eliminating trigger points.

In some patients suffering from severe RSD (such as causalgia), repetitive injections of the trigger point may be done by the patient through a subcutaneous catheter.[199]

HOT TRIGGER POINT INJECTION

Infrequently the trigger point may be hot rather than cold on thermography. It is usually due to injury to the articular facets of the spine as well as muscular ligamentous or neural injury in soft tissues surrounding the spine (Figure 2a).

CHEMICAL SYMPATHETIC NERVE BLOCK

Chemical sympathetic nerve block is done in presynaptic (central α- and β-receptor block) and peripheral receptor blocks.

PRESYNAPTIC β CHEMICAL BLOCK

Presynaptic B chemical block is achieved by β-receptor blockers such as propranolol (Inderal) and by calcium channel blockers.

β-BLOCKERS

This form of treatment decreases the β-adrenergic response and thus helps the central origin types of RSDs such as migraine and other forms of atypical face pain of central origin. β block with propranolol has a series of side effects such as hypotension, bradycardia, depression,

TABLE 20
Commonly Used Sympathetic Blockers

α-Blockers	β-blockers	Calcium influx blockers[a]	Presynaptic (brain stem) blockers[a]
α$_1$-Blocker			
Phenoxybenzamine (Dibenzyline)[a]	Timolol (Blockadrene)	Nifedipine (Procardia)	Clonidine-hydrochloride[b] (Catapres)
Terazocin[a] (Hytrin)			
Prozacin[a] (Minipres)	Propranolol[b] (Inderal)	Diltiazem (Cardizem)	Propranolol[b] (Inderal)
α$_2$-Blocker	Atenolol (Tenormin)	Verapamil (Calan)	
Yohimbine[c]		Nicardepene (Cardene)	
Idazoxan[566]			

[a] First choice should be phenoxybenzamine, Terazocin, or Prozacin. If they do not work, then others may be tried. This is an exclusive α$_1$-adrenergic receptors' supersensitivity.[509,510]

[b] The disruption of efferent sympathetic modulation results in supersensitivity of sensory end organs to norepinephrine.[509] Excessive efferent sympathetic modulation (RSD) activates the α$_1$ sensory receptors. So, α$_1$-blockers are quite effective in control of RSD. The β-blockers and presynaptic blockers are not as helpful.

[c] Yohimbine[559–565] 5.4 mg five times a day is well tolerated and a good adjunct in treatment of RSD. It is a presynaptic α$_2$-blocker.

TABLE 21
Side Effects of Propranolol

Depression
Fatigue
Decreased libido
Decreased sexual function
Irritability
Sleep disorder
Difficulty concentrating
Disturbance of recent memory
A form of hangover headache

fatigue, weakness of myocardium, hypotension, aggravation of cardiac arrhythmias, and aggravation of asthma. Sudden withdrawal can cause supersensitivity to catecholamines with resultant cardiac arrhythmias and myocardial infarction. Whereas propranolol is a peripheral β$_1$- and β$_2$-adrenergic blocker, it also has CNA effects of drowsiness and depression when administered in high doses (see Cecil *Textbook of Medicine*). Propranolol has been used in neurology for management of tremor, migraine headaches, RSD, and bursts of agressive behavior in children and teenagers.[10,70]

It is well known that propranolol has an exclusive β-adrenergic blocking effect peripherally. On the other hand, β-adrenergic blockers do not block discharges produced by sympathetic stimulation in peripheral neuromas.[82,395]

Propranolol blocks the β-adrenergic receptors in the brain, especially in the brain stem. In this regard, the brain stem receptors in effect are "peripheral" receptors for the β-adrenergic system.

The β-adrenergic blocking agents are either fat soluble or water soluble. The most fat-soluble β-adrenergic blocking agent is propranolol. Due to the fact that it is a fat-soluble agent, it exerts a significant influence on CNS function.

Conant et al.[66] summarized the CNS side effects of propranolol and atenolol. They studied the undesirable effects of propranolol on CNS in the form of depression and other CNS unwanted effects of this agent. These are summarized in Table 21.

Their study concluded that atenolol, which is more water soluble, has far less side effects than propranolol.

Patten[266] carried out a detailed review of the depressive effects of propranolol on the CNS: "Propranolol was found to cause depression as a side effect with a statistically greater frequency than the control medications used in these trials. As other side effects of propranolol included fatigue, diminished energy, decreased libido, anorexia, and poor concentration, it is suggested that propranolol is a cause of organic mood disorder, depressed type."[266]

Other reports[108,120,218,266,268,278,284,357] confirm similar side effects of propranolol. Golden et al.[115] emphasized the serious side effects of propranolol withdrawal. Specifically, psychosis may result from such withdrawal.[115,267] Other serious complications of sudden propranolol withdrawal include myocardial ischemia and infarction, unstable angina, ventricular tachycardia, severe tremor, diaphoresis, and malaise.[267]

Realizing that symptoms such as migraine headache and tremor are quite common among alcohol abusers, and realizing that it is difficult to make the diagnosis of closet drinkers who have such complications, propranolol should not be used in such patients. Its use in alcohol abusers not only aggravates depression, but also exacerbates orthostatic hypotension.

The use of propranolol in high doses (up to 320 mg/day) has been reported beneficial in isolated cases of causalgias.[199,276,341] On the other hand, a double blind crossover trial of propranolol in such patients stressed no relief of pain.[318]

In general, the use of **propranolol** should be discouraged in patients suffering from RSD. The only exceptions are severe migraine due to RSD and cases of RSD that are accompanied by **coronary artery disease**.[9] Even then, the use of **procardia** (Nifedipin) or **calcium channel blockers** is preferred.

α₂-BLOCKER

Yohimbine[559–565] is effective in blocking α_2-receptors and increases the circulation in genitalia and extremities. It is well tolerated. It increases the circulation in extremities as well as in genitalia. The usual dose is 5.4 mg four to five times a day.

CALCIUM CHANNEL BLOCKERS

Calcium channel blockers[205,283,365] such as nifedipin (Procardia and Cardene) relax smooth muscles, increase peripheral blood flow, and counteract the effect of norepinephrin on blood vessels. Such blockers also suppress abnormal calcium conductance at areas of nerve degeneration in ephaptic scars.[80] Nifedipin given 10 to 30 mg tid resulted in complete relief of pain in 7 of 11 causalgic patients.[280] It is well tolerated by RSD patients.

CENTRAL α-RECEPTOR CHEMICAL BLOCKERS

The next form of presynaptic blockage is achieved by stimulation of α-receptors in brain stem with resultant decrease of sympathetic outflow. This is done with the help of clonidine (catapres). It is quite a helpful treatment in doses as much as 0.1 to 0.2 mg up to three times a day. However, it has its own side effects in the form of postural hypotension, insomnia, and depression.

PERIPHERAL α₁-RECEPTOR CHEMICAL BLOCKERS

Peripheral α_1-blockers are the blockers of choice for treatment of RSD. These blockers should be considered the first to use in RSD patients.

This is achieved by the use of phenoxybenzamine (Dibenzyline).[62] This is quite a potent α_1-receptor blocker. It was used on a series of soldiers in the Lebanese War. The results have been quite impressive; but because it is a strong α-receptor blocker, it has its own side effects. Usually the dosage starts at 10 mg at bed time with very gradual increase to no more than 10 mg tid. Ghostin et al.[62] report practically 100% relief after 6 to 12 weeks of treatment in causalgias secondary to battlefield missiles with a dose of 40 to 120 mg/day. These results are practically impossible to replicate in causalgic patients: the high dosage of 40 to 120 mg/day is fraught with dizziness secondary to hypotension. Somehow, as is the case with sympathectomy

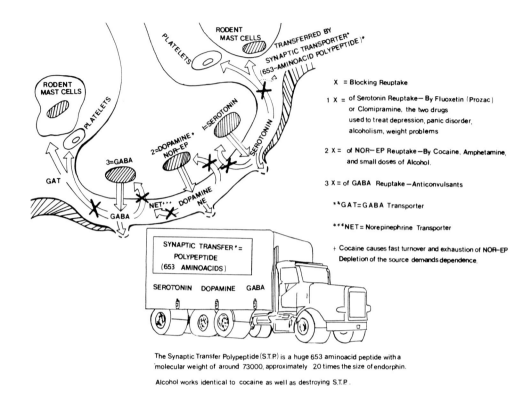

X = Blocking Reuptake

1 X = of Serotonin Reuptake— By Fluoxetin (Prozac) or Clomipramine, the two drugs used to treat depression, panic disorder, alcoholism, weight problems

2 X = of NOR–EP Reuptake—By Cocaine, Amphetamine, and small doses of Alcohol.

3 X = of GABA Reuptake —Anticonvulsants

**GAT=GABA Transporter

***NET= Norepinephrine Transporter

+ Cocaine causes fast turnover and exhaustion of NOR–EP Depletion of the source demands dependence.

SYNAPTIC TRANSFER * = POLYPEPTIDE (653 AMINOACIDS)

SEROTONIN   DOPAMINE   GABA

The Synaptic Transfer Polypeptide (S.T.P.) is a huge 653 aminoacid peptide with a molecular weight of around 73000, approximately 20 times the size of endorphin.

Alcohol works identical to cocaine as well as destroying S.T.P.

FIGURE 28. The synaptic transfer protein (STP)[479] is a large protein made of 653 amino acids (20 times larger than ACTH and over 100 times larger than endorphin) essential in transfer and restorage of the neurotransmitters from synapse back to presynaptic neuron as well as rodent mast cells and to platelets. Any chemical (e.g., ETOH) that disrupts its function disrupts the supply of neurotransmitters. ETOH causes the death of nerve cells and destruction of STP.

for battlefield causalgias, the 100% relief from such treatments cannot be replicated in civil injuries.

Prazosin (Minipres), another α-blocker, given to the patient at 2 mg/day by mouth twice a day, has resulted in good relief in causalgia.[2] The side effects consist of postural hypotension, tachycardia, poor ejaculation, myosis, and nasal congestion. The dizziness (hypotension) and weakness make it impractical to use this drug in a majority of patients.

Terazocin (Hytrin) is a very well-tolerated α-blocker. If the patient cannot tolerate the above two α-blockers, Terazocin can be an excellent substitute.

TRANSCUTANEOUS ELECTRICAL NERVE STIMULATOR (TNS)

TNS is quite helpful in disuse dystrophy. In case of ephaptic dystrophy, TNS should not be applied to the scar area, but its application to the proximal area of the extremity can be beneficial. However, application of TNS to the trigger points is quite effective in control of pain. TNS has been reported to be quite effective in pediatric RSD.[339]

TNS has an advantage over invasive stimulation (e.g., epidural, thalamic, or periaqueductal stimulation): it can be stopped and restarted in a **noninvasive** fashion.

The **invasive devices** are usually successful in the first 9 to 18 months. After 1.5 years the brain ignores the digital stimulation of the invasive stimulators, and the devices become useless for relief of pain.

DIET

Modern medicine relies mainly on the application of drugs and surgery to cure all ills.

There is no difference between drugs and food. The first lesson in toxicology is that the difference between food, drugs, and poisons is only a matter of dosage and quantity.

Any chemical formed in nature uninfluenced by civilized humans can be considered a food, if edible. Any chemical composed by humans in a laboratory is more likely to be a drug than a food.

Even the nutrients added to intravenous fluids and nasogastric tubings to supplement nutrition in the long run result in malnutrition due to the lack of trace chemicals essential for proper nutrition.

For decades physicians have ignored, ridiculed, and underestimated proper nutrition and dietary habits. The dietary revolution in the past 30 years started by the hippies in California drastically reduced the incidence of stroke and heart attack. Only in the past 8 to 10 years have reputable medical journals published articles on the subject of food as preventive medicine against cancer and heart attack.

The physician prescribes a few miligrams of certain medicines for the patient and considers it a cure for his or her illness. The relatives of the patient, TV hype, and chiropractors convince the patient not to take medicine. On the other hand, the chemicals in the food continue to destroy the patient's health.

Even some of the drugs classified as food by the government, e.g., beer, are consumed by the patient even if she is pregnant and her future child may most likely end up suffering from fetal alcohol syndrome (FAS).[481] The drinking father may contribute to FAS as well. In our study of 22 classic FAS children, 4 were the product of a tee-totaler mother and alcoholic father.

FOOD AS A STIMULANT

The protein in food breaks down into amino acids that influence the cerebral function (Figure 29).

There are two main groups of protein in food. One group is a stimulant represented by the amino acid **tyrosine** (Figure 29), which is mainly present in red meat, red wine, and sharp cheese. As seen in figure 29, the tyrosine is the precursor of **catecholamine**. The catecholamine receptors in the brain, especially in the brain stem, are the key to the state of alertness, arousal, and hyperexcitability. **Cocaine**, by increasing the release of catecholamines into these receptors and stimulating the formation and breakdown of catecholamines, causes excitation, lack of sleep, feelings of omnipotence, as well as agitation and restlessness. This increased turnover and breakdown of catecholamines result in depletion of the vital biogenic amines (catechols) and may cause severe withdrawal. Similar effects may be noted with the use of small doses of alcohol or the use of coffee or chocolate (which contains theobromine, caffeine, and phenethylamine).

A diet high in tyrosine has an effect similar to that of the above-mentioned drugs.

The second group of proteins in food has a calming effect opposite to tyrosine. The common denominator in this group is **tryptophan**, which is rich in yogurt, mild cheese, and **4-F diet** (fresh fruit, fresh vegetable, fish, and fowl) (Table 22). Tryptophan, as seen in Table 23, is the precursor for serotonin. The ubiquitous serotonin is the common denominator for counteracting pain, especially headache, insomnia, agitation, and depressive agitation.

What differentiates a lion from a lamb is the tyrosine-rich diet vs. the tryptophan-rich diet. Stated a different way, it is the difference between a meat eater and a vegetarian.

DIET AND RSD

In RSD the tyrosine-dopamine-norepinephrine system is in full swing. The patient should ideally become a vegetarian to counteract the hyperactive dopamine system with the help of tryptophan-generated serotonin.

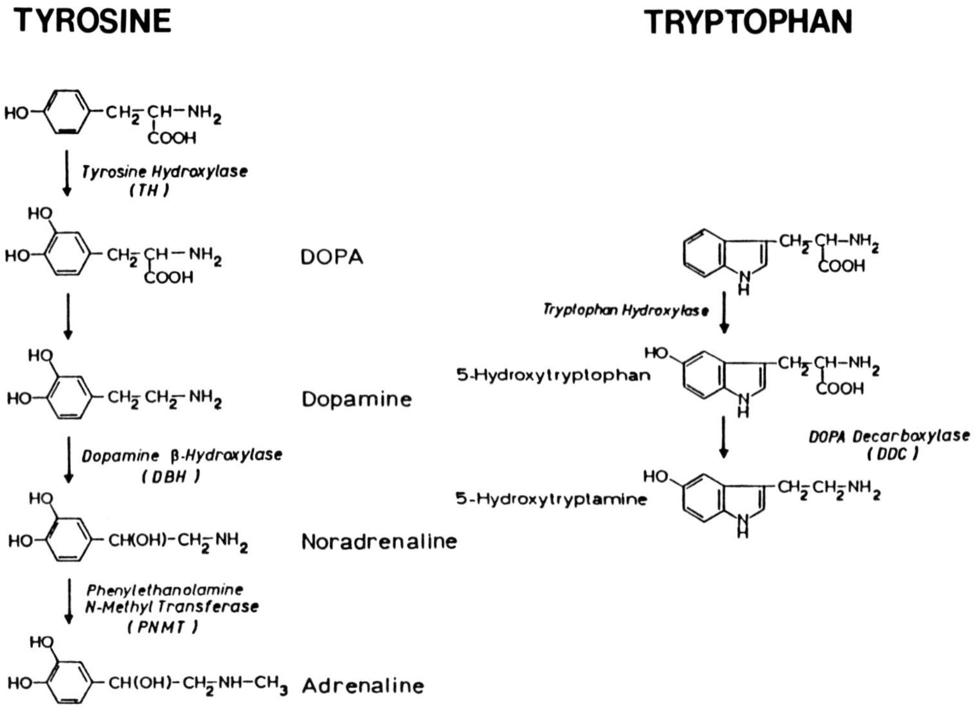

TYROSINE   **TRYPTOPHAN**

HO—⟨ ⟩—CH₂-CH—NH₂ / COOH

↓ *Tyrosine Hydroxylase (TH)*

HO, HO—⟨ ⟩—CH₂-CH—NH₂ / COOH   DOPA

CH₂-CH—NH₂ / COOH

Tryptophan Hydroxylase ↓

↓

HO, HO—⟨ ⟩—CH₂ CH₂—NH₂   Dopamine

5-Hydroxytryptophan   HO—⟨ ⟩—CH₂-CH—NH₂ / COOH

↓ *Dopamine β-Hydroxylase (DBH)*

DOPA Decarboxylase (DDC) ↓

HO, HO—⟨ ⟩—CH(OH)-CH₂—NH₂   Noradrenaline

5-Hydroxytryptamine   HO—⟨ ⟩—CH₂ CH₂ NH₂

↓ *Phenylethanolamine N-Methyl Transferase (PNMT)*

HO, HO—⟨ ⟩—CH(OH)-CH₂-NH—CH₃   Adrenaline

FIGURE 29. Tyrosine and trytophan are the two leading and opposing amino acids in food. Tyrosine is the precursor of dopamine and norepinephrine, hence, a stimulator of behavior. Tryptophan is the precursor of 5-HT and serotonin, hence, an antidepressant and moderator of behavior. Mild cheese, similar to fish and foul, is rich in tryptophan. Sharp cheese, similar to red meat, is rich in tyrosine.

As is the case with other forms of chronic pain, without application of proper diet, the rate of success in the treatment of RSD is going to be quite low.

On top of the list of things to be avoided in a diet are any chemicals that stimulate the formation of catecholamines. These consist of alcohol, chocolate, hot dogs, cold cuts, and red meat. These chemicals are deleterious to RSD because of a rise in tyrosine as well as introduction of chemicals such as nitrites and alcohol with the tendency to raise the level of catecholamine and norepinephrine in the brain.

Diet without exercise is practically useless.[133,423]

The diet shown in Table 22 is helpful in the treatment of RSD, migraine headache, migraine in children, and attention deficit in children. It is based on intake of foods rich in tryptophan and fructose and low in tyrosine and sucrose. It also eliminates stimulants such as chocolate (containing phenethylamine, which is a strong stimulant) and caffeine. It eliminates hot dogs (containing nitrites), cold cuts (containing strong chemical preservatives), and excessive intake of the five "C"s (candy, cookies, chocolate, cake, and cocktails). RSD is simply a hyperactive norepinephrine state. It makes no sense to apply sympatholytic medications to patients and to allow them to eat foods rich in tyrosine. Tyrosine as a precursor to norepinephrine stimulates the sympathetic system.

The main principle of a diet for RSD, chronic pain, or headache is a diet rich in tryptophan and low in tyrosine. Tryptophan raises the CNS level of serotonin, whereas tyrosine raises the level of dopamine and norepinephrine (Figure 29).

A surge of tyrosine in the diet (e.g., port wine, red meat, and sharp cheese) stimulates formation of dopamine and epinephrine. The secondary stimulation of insulin results in reactive hypoglycemia and lowered threshold for pain. Foods rich in tryptophan (e.g., mild cheese, white meat, and yogurt) exert an opposite effect.

TABLE 22
Neurological Associates Four F's Diet (H. Hooshmand, M.D.)

The four F's:
1. Fresh Fruit — not canned
2. Fresh vegetables — Olive oil is the best cooking oil
3. Fish — baked or broiled. Use fresh lemon juice for flavor. Avoid the use of margarine
4. Fowl — skinned! not fried — baked, roasted or grilled is fine. When you are in a hurry, try wrapping a boneless breast with vegetables (i.e., onions and bell peppers) in aluminum foil and baking — it is quick and easy

Avoid the five C's: cookies, cakes, chocolate, cocktails, and candy

Foods to be avoided

Crystalline sugar
Soft drinks with sugar
Pies
Bologna
Salami
Hot dogs
Sherbet
Ice cream
Enriched white flour
 (bleached flour)
Syrups
Mayonnaise
White bread
All fried foods
Canned fruits packed in syrup

Cakes
Sweetrolls
Lard
Crisco and other shortenings
 (replace with olive oil)
Potato chips
Dips
Cake mixes
Alcohol
Nondairy cream substitutes
Margarine
Donuts
Butter
Bacon and any pork
Candies

Foods allowed rarely or sparingly
No Coffee (may be replaced with iced tea)
Lamb
Tea
Pulp of potato (may fry in olive oil)

Foods that are allowed
Diet drinks — no caffeine, sugar, and low to no sodium
Skim cheese
Apples
All fresh fruit
Unsweetened orange juice
Natural fresh-squeezed orange juice and grapefruit juice
Apple juice — no added sugar, natural
All fresh vegetables
Veal
Chicken and other fowl — skinned
Lobster (no butter)
Lean roast beef (in moderation)
Raisins
Skim milk
Tuna (water-packed)
Nuts — raw and unsalted
Honey — natural
Oatmeal (plain and unflavored)
Lowfat cottage cheese
Lowfat plain yogurt — flavored has sugar — add your own fresh fruit
Sweet potato with skin
Eggs — no more than two/week
Sardines
All fish
Cereals — whole grain, low sugar
Shrimp

TABLE 22 (Continued)
Neurological Associates Four F's Diet (H. Hooshmand, M.D.)

Fruits — dried
Crab

Drink 6–8 glasses of water per day

Labels — read them! Be aware of the word "carbohydrates". Frequently it is a euphemism for sugar. Be aware of the ratio of fat to calories. Avoid high fat to calories ratios. Also, high cholesterol and preservatives/chemicals (or flavorings) should be avoided. An ingredients list that is very long and has many unrecognizable (unpronounceable) words should also be avoided. Remember very low to no added salt

Food preparation — Avoid adding fats (oil, margarine, etc.) and salt during and after preparation. Try to prepare in ways that do not require oil/fat — such as steam, back, broil, roast. Definitely *do not fry*!!! (Olive oil is okay)

Salad Bars — The tendency to eat free food results in excessive calories! Therefore, it is for this reason that salad bars can be deceptive. They seem to be more of a high calorie/fat, all you can eat buffet. When confronted with one, stick to the fresh fruits and vegetables — *avoid* the desserts (i.e., puddings, cakes, etc.)

Diet fads
"Cheese is rich in cholesterol". There are two types of cheese: sharp cheese rich in tyrosine is harmful to RSD patients; mild cheese (e.g., mozarella, ricotta, muenster) contains only 25–30 mg cholesterol per serving (in contrast to liver, 375 mg, and kielbasa, 400 mg)
"Shell fish has too much cholesterol". Shellfish contains HDL cholesterol, which is preventive against any form of vascular disease
"Don't eat food before going to sleep". Wrong: Don't consume red meat, coffee, or chocolate. Eating fruits and dairy products before bedtime is quite helpful in chronic pain (such as RSD)

Coffee
Coffee should be avoided altogether in patients suffering from RSD; to consider coffee as a simple conveyor of caffeine is naive
1.   Coffee has an acid-based oil that is an irritant to gastric mucosa. It stimulates the secretion of gastric acidity. Secondarily, the high gastric acidity results in secretion of adrenalin. The secretion of adrenalin stimulates insulin secretion with resultant secondary relative hypoglycemia. The end result is tension, a mild rise in blood pressure, and 2-3 hours later craving sweets because of the relative hypoglycemia.
       Obviously none of the above is helpful in RSD. The rise in plasma epinephrine will undo whatever good medications are doing to counteract the hyperactive dopaminergic system in RSD.
2.   Coffee is more harmful than caffeinated soft drinks or tea
3.   Mild tea does not cause reactive hypoglycemia and a rise in blood pressure
4.   Tea, if prepared in mild form (not too strong), contains less caffeine. It has no acid-based oil as does coffee. It contains tannin. Tannin or tannic acid curbs thirst and results in less demand for further consumption of tea or coffee
5.   Coffee and tea both temporarily raise the body temperature. A few minutes after drinking coffee, the stimulation of the dopaminergic system causes colder extremities and a simultaneous rise in systemic temperature. Tea has a much milder effect in this regard. The cold extremities aggravate RSD
6.   Iced tea seems to be the mildest and the safest of caffeinated drinks
7.   A patient with high fever is harmed by coffee and helped by tea and lemon juice. As is the case with home-made chicken soup being helpful to the sick (in contrast with factory-made red meat type of soup) for unknown reasons, mild tea has a healing effect, and coffee has an aggravating effect in patients suffering from stress and fever, including stress of complex chronic pain

Herbal tea
Just because tea is less harmful than coffee does not imply that herbal tea is good or healthy for anyone. Herbal teas are a variety of different dried vegetable leaves. Some of the herbs contain toxic substances that are harmful to anyone — including RSD patients. Because of the variety in strength and quality of chemicals in herbs, the use of herbal teas should be avoided. Some of them contain such high doses of tannins (e.g., sassafras tea) that can be carcinogenic. Catnip, juniper, nutmet, and hydrangia may be hallucinogenic. Chamomile and marigold may be fatally allergenic. Senna leaves, aloe leaves, and duck roots can be strongly cathartic. Mistletoe leaves and horsetail grass may cause fatal toxicity. So why bother with such chemicals?

TABLE 23
Food and Stress

	Eustress	Distress
Diet type	4F: lactovegetarian and seafood	Diet rich in red meat
Fats	Monounsaturated (e.g., olive oil)	Saturated (e.g., fat in red meat)
Cholesterol	HDL (fish oil)	LDL (animal fat)
Amino acids (protein)	Tryptophan (mild cheese, yogurt, fish, and fowl)	Tyrosine (sharp cheese, red meat)
Carbohydrates	Complex (rice, pasta, and fructose)	Crystalline sugar (sucrose)
Alcohol	Maximum 1 oz per day: most people cannot stop at that, so abstain	Over 2 drinks per day

TABLE 24
Some Hormones and Neurotransmitters in Brain Stem and Limbic System

	Nucleus raphe obscurus	Nucleus raphe pallidus	Nucleus raphe magnus	Nucleus raphe pontis	Nucleus raphe dorsalis	Nucleus raphe superior	Nucleus raphe oralis
Serotonin	+	+	+	+	+	+	+
ACTH					+		
GABA					+		
CCK			+				
β-Endorphin				+			
LHRH			+	+	+	+	+
leu-ENK		+		+	+	+	
met-ENK		+		+	+	+	
α-MSH					+		
Substance P	+	+	+	+	+	+	+

Abstracted from Emson.[92]

The key note in an RSD diet is avoidance of distress with the help of 4-F (fresh fruit, fresh vegetables, fish, and foul). The emphasis is on fresh to avoid superoxide transformation, to avoid release of rogue oxygen, and to **avoid peroxidation** (H_2O + rogue oxygen → H_2O_2) and further destruction of the pathologic lesions in RSD.

ALCOHOL AND SMOKING

Alcohol (also see Alcohol Abuse and RSD in Chapter 9) is a dilator of surface vessels in the skin, but it constricts muscular (heart and other muscles) and soft tissue arterioles. It has a deleterious effect on RSD due to both vascular effect and aggravation of pain as a CNS depressant (see chapter on Alcohol and RSD).

Cigarette smoking has been found to be almost twice as common in RSD patients (68 vs. 37%) as in hospitalized controls.[212] As with alcohol, it aggravates RSD in multiple modes, not the least being its effect in replacing oxygen with carbon monoxide with secondary hypoxic effect.

HORMONE TREATMENT: ADRENOCORTICOIDS (LAZAROIDS)

RSD is a chronic illness. Long-term use of lazaroids (cortisone, prednisone, and dexamethasone) in RSD is of no use.

Except for postherpetic neuralgia in acute stage, the use of adrenocorticosteroids (such as

TABLE 25
ACTH Application in Neurology

Pituitary insufficiency[a]
Lennox Gastaunt epilepsy in retarded infants[a]
   (Trojaborg,[574] Bower[549])
Multiple sclerosis[a]
Chronic pain[a] (Hooshmand et al.[147])
Cigarette addiction[a] (Bourne,[554] West[555])
Anorexia nervosa[a]

[a]   Adrenal steroids not effective.

long-term treatment of RSD) can cause serious side effects (e.g., adrenal atrophy, depression, and orthostatic hypotension).

NARCOTICS AND CHRONIC PAIN OF RSD

The management of acute vs. chronic pain requires a completely opposite approach. Whereas in severe acute pain the use of narcotics is vital and essential, in chronic pain application of narcotics is contraindicated and dangerous.

Approaches such as the use of Dilaulid as a focal perfusate in the RSD extremity make no sense. Although the narcotic results in immediate relief of pain it is followed by an exaggerated painful withdrawal.

Oral or intramuscular (i.m.) application of narcotics flood the CNS with resultant inhibition of endorphin formation followed by severe pain of withdrawal.

For the purpose of lasting analgesia — in chronic pain of RSD — the CNS should be stimulated to form more endorphins. The use of narcotics results in a marked inhibition and reduction of endorphins. Exercise and proper nutrition stimulate the formation of endorphins.

The chemical treatment of choice for chronic pain of RSD is antidepressants or ACTH, both of which raise the concentration of endorphins in CNS.

ACTH AND ENDORPHINS

ACTH and endorphins have a common percursor called proopiomelanocortin. The neurotransmitter 5-hydroxytryptamine (5H-T) is the originator of cholecystokinin (CCK), TRH, and corticotrophin-releasing factor (CRF). The CRF or proopiomelanocortin releases not only ACTH but at least 17 other hormones and neurotransmitters. The function of only a few of these neurotransmitters has been recognized. These are ACTH, endorphins, and melanocyte-stimulating hormone (MSH) (see Table 26).

The proopiomelanocortin (POMC) (Figures 30 and 31) normally produces endorphin, MSH, and ACTH according to the peripheral demand regulated by hypothalamus.

With the use of exorphins (narcotics), the POMC reduces its production of endorophins because of lack of peripheral demand, and, in turn, increases the formation of ACTH and MSH (Figure 32).

With the use of **exogenous ACTH** (i.m. or i.v.), the **POMC reduces its formation of ACTH** and **generates more endorphins and MSH**.

It becomes obvious that in patients who are dependent on large doses of narcotics, the use of **i.m. or i.v. ACTH increases the formation of endorphins**.

Hughes and Kosterlitz in 1975 extracted leu-met-enkephalin (LMENK) from a pig's brain.

Mains et al. in 1977 demonstrated that POMC is richly concentrated in the hypothalamus, especially in the infundibular region of the periaqueductal gray. In the same area, this large protein precursor is cleaved into ACTH, MSH, or β-endorphins depending on demand.

TABLE 26
ACTH

	Ref.
Prevents cyclophosphamide (750 mg/surface meter) and Cisplastin (75 mg/surface meter) Toxic neuropathy	387
Cerebral ACTH Loci	92
1. Nucleus raphe dorsalis of brain stem 2. Hippocampus 3. Arcuate (infundibular) nucleus Surrounding infundibulum of 3rd ventricle High concentration of POMC, ACTH, MSH, β-endorphin	
Hormones affecting ACTH	
Naltroxene and naloxone Increase ACTH, cortisol and LHRH: decrease GH	550, 551
POMC	
Peptide, ACTH, α-MSH, and β-endorphins are present in the same areas of hypothalamic cells and are secreted by a common precursor prooptiocortin 31k substance	552

ACTH, MSH, and endorphins are present in other areas of the brain simultaneously in a group or individually.

The areas that show concentration of the above hormones and neurotransmitters along with concentration of substance P include nucleus cuneiformis, reticular formation of brain stem, hippocampal region, and the periaqueductal gray.[30,31,140,160,164,198,270,271,347,400]

It is obvious that **ACTH** has nothing in common with corticosteroids except that it **stimulates the formation of the natural corticosteroids** (Figures 30 and 31).

ACTH is effective in treatmenxt of chronic pain that is perpetuated by the use of narcotics.

In our experience[150] the use of **i.v. ACTH** from 1982 through 1986 **shortened hospital stays** for detoxification from narcotics on an average of 8 days.

The placebo group detoxification patients who were treated with standard detoxification treatment were hospitalized an average of 17 days in contrast to 9 days for the ACTH group: the range was 6 to 25 days for the non-ACTH group and 6 to 15 days for the ACTH group.

ACTH was least effective in ephaptic dystrophy (six cases with an average hospital stay of 15 days) and **most effective in other types of pain** (average hospital stay 7 days).

Reid et al.[293] and Stubbs et al.[358] demonstrated the **reduction of ACTH** and endorphins as well as reduction of **leutinizing hormone** (LH) and **follicle-stimulating hormone** (FSH) in patients who were treated with **exorphins** (narcotics).

Vanderhoop et al.[387] demonstrated the beneficial effect of ACTH in prevention of toxic peripheral neuropathy due to cyclophosphamide and cisplastin.

It is concluded that when the patient has suffered from chronic pain and has been on narcotics, the use of **ACTH enhances the formation of endorphins from POMC**. In this regard, it is quite **helpful in treatment of chronic pain** (Figure 32).

ENDORPHINS AND SNS

Endorphins play a major role in the descending inhibitory system for the modulation of pain. They are abundant in the brain stem and spinal cord and they are present in the fibers and a few ganglion cell bodies in the sympathetic ganglia.[474]

A. CORTISOL

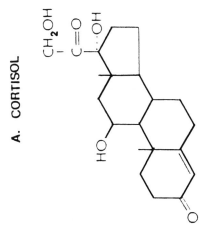

B. ACTH

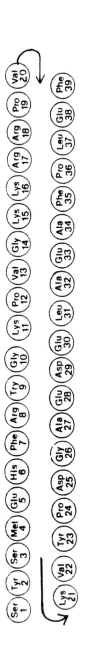

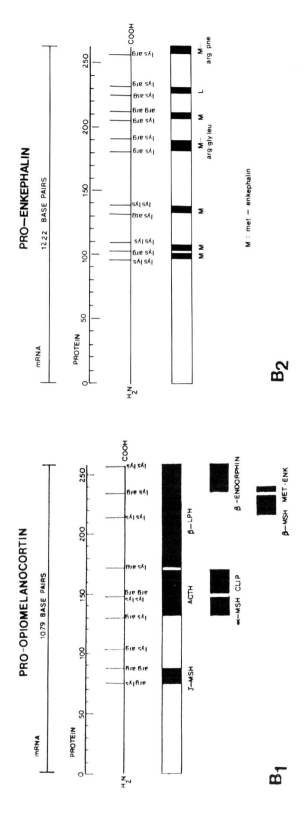

FIGURE 30. ACTH is not a corticosteroid. It is cleaved from proopiomelanocortin (POMC). The POMC is 1079 base pairs in RNA. It is the precursor of 39-amino acid ACTH. It also produces MSH and endorphins (Figure 31).

Morphine, Endorphins, and Naloxone

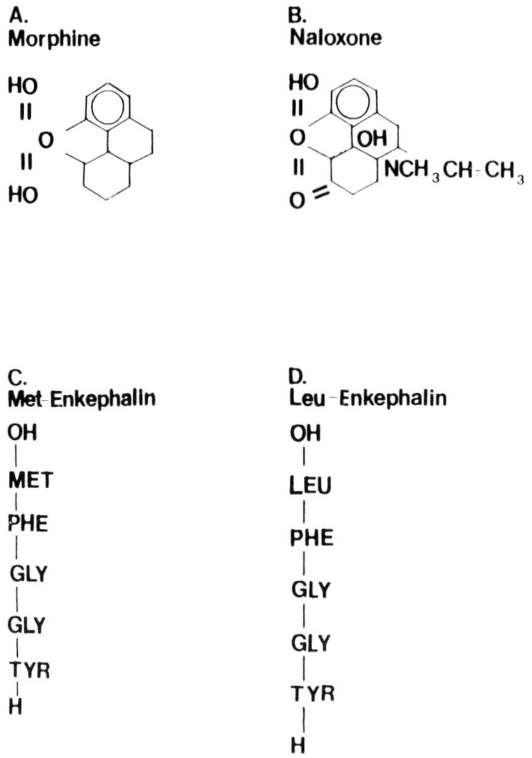

A.
Morphine

HO
$\parallel$
O
$\parallel$
HO

B.
Naloxone

HO
$\parallel$
O   OH
$\parallel$ $NCH_3CH\text{-}CH_3$
O

C.
Met-Enkephalin

OH
|
MET
|
PHE
|
GLY
|
GLY
|
TYR
|
H

D.
Leu-Enkephalin

OH
|
LEU
|
PHE
|
GLY
|
GLY
|
TYR
|
H

FIGURE 31. The enkephalins are 5-amino acid peptide hormones with a stronger narcotic effect than the synthetic morphine (exorphin).

Although the opiate peptide, enkephalin, has an affinity for cholinergic structures, it is also present in the paravertebral sympathetic ganglia.[474] Animal studies reveal a tapering down of endorphins from the CNS to sympathetic ganglia, and a coexistence of substance P (sP) with endorphins in the same ganglia. This suggests an excitatory-inhibitory balance between sP and endorphins.

Dynorphins are present in higher concentrations in the sympathetic ganglia, spinal cord gray matter than in the brain stem region. This may suggest a supplemental inhibitory role for dynorphins in the spinal cord.

Endorphins are plentiful in the hypothalamic region and the limbic system, suggesting that endorphins have a role in behavior.

Injection of opiate peptides in the CSF results in dramatic alterations in animal behavior.[475] Hooshmand et al.[150] have shown a reduction of endorphins in CSF of chronic pain patients.

ACTH IN NEUROPSYCHIATRIC DISORDERS

Studies regarding pharmacology, immunochemistry, and histochemistry of ACTH reveal that ACTH is present in the pituitary gland and in other areas of the brain such as the brain stem and hypothalamus. ACTH-containing fibers are seen in the cortex of the cerebral hemispheres as well as nucleus raphe dorsalis in the brain stem and periaqueductal central gray matter.[412]

Immunocytochemical studies demonstrate the presence of ACTH and endorphins in common sites as in the sites outlined above. A chemical study of structures of ACTH, MSH, and

PROPOSED MECHANISM OF ACTION
OF ACTH IN CHRONIC PAIN

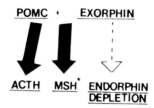

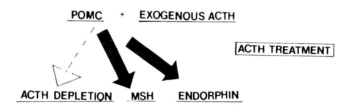

ACTH, a byproduct of (POMC) pro-opiomelanocortin which
also produces endorphin & MSH.

ACTH increases the concentration of beta endorphin
in CSF (Hooshmand): A reflection of increased formation
of endorphin.

ACTH acts as an antagonist of the analgesic effect
of beta endorphin (Mains, et al, 1977)
˙ One typical give-away sign of opium addicts is an
acquired dark skin.

FIGURE 32. Proposed mechanism of action of ACTH. POMC breaks down to ACTH, MSH, endorphin, and other byproducts. With application of exorphins, the endorphins are depleted. The reverse occurs with the application of exogenous ACTH. The endogenous ACTH becomes depleted with resultant increase in the formation of MSH and endorphin. ACTH is a byproduct of proopiomelanocortin (POMC), which also produces endorphin and MSH. ACTH increases the concentration of β-endorphin in CSF (Hooshmand), a reflection of increased formation of endorphin. ACTH acts as an antagonist of the analgesic effect of β-endorphin (Mains et al., 1977). *One typical sign of opium addicts is an acquired dark skin.

TABLE 27
Intravenous ACTH in Chronic Pain, 1982–1986

ACTH (23 cases)	No ACTH (24 cases)
Hospital days	
Average	
9	17
Range	
6–15	6–25

Effect of intravenous ACTH on length of hospitalization for chronic pain
Ephaptic RSD causalgia (6 cases)

Average stay	15 days
Detoxification (4 cases)	
Average stay	7 days

TABLE 28
Modes of Therapy

80 units ACTH in 250 ml D5 and W through i.v. heparin lock to run in 3 hours/day for 7 days
Outpatient method: 40 units ACTH gel i.m. 3–4 times a week for 12 weeks

Precaution: Zantac or Tagamet on daily basis should be given to prevent gastric irritation

The above doses should be individualized and adjusted according to the patient's tolerance: if water retention, depression, or skin infection (furoncles) develops, the dose should be reduced and spaced out. By and large, outpatient i.m. ACTH is better tolerated than the i.v. dose.

TABLE 29
Plasma ACTH

	Chronic pain[a]	Acute pain[b]
Plasma ACTH (pg/ml)	62–80	69–103
CSF ACTH (pg/ml)	91–101	97–103

[a]   Negative myelogram in eight patients with over 6 months pain.
[b]   Acute disc herniation in myelograms of eight patients with less than 2 months pain.

TABLE 30
ACTH and Depression: Incidence of Depression
(MMPI, Millon Tests)

	Patients	Percent
Prior to treatment	68	82
After ACTH treatment	31	74
After treatment with other methods	32	78

	Follow-up after 4 years	
	ACTH group	Non-ACTH group
Less pain	27 (65%)	20 (49%)
No change	14 (33%	19 (46%)
More pain	1 (2.4%)	2 (4.8%)
Return to narcotics	7 (16%)	11 (26%)

TABLE 31
Endorphins[a]

	Endorphins[476–479,556] (enkephalins, dynorphin)	Exorphins
Pain relief	Yes	Yes
Antidepressant	Yes	No
Strength	100 × stronger	100 × weaker
Dose release	Microjet	Flooding dosage
Effect on other hormones	Stimulate sex hormones, thyroid hormone	Block secretion of hormones
"Acid rain" effect[b]	No	Yes: flooding the brain temporarily leaving the brain devoid of hormones on withdrawal
Appetite	Increased	Reduced
Sex desire	Increased	Reduced
REM sleep		
Quality of sleep	Increased	Reduced
Duration of effect	Very brief with no significant withdrawal	Prolonged with drastic withdrawal
Sympathetic function	Reduced: warm extremities and normalized BP	Increased during withdrawal: cold extremities, hypertension follows initial hypotension
Effect on endo-BZs	Stimulate more BZs resulting in tranquility	Inhibit ENDO-BZs resulting in withdrawal: anxiety, agitation
Effect on sex hormones and steroids	Increased	Markedly reduced
Effect on limbic system	Stimulate and normalize: better sleep, better memory, better judgment	Inhibit and flood the system: insomnia amnesia poor judgment
Tolerance	Not known	Strong[c]

[a] There are two types of cells in the brain. The nerves, and the glial cells protecting the nerves. The nerves secrete hormones. The glial cells don't. The brain is an endocrine gland-controlling behavior with secretion of hormones. Endorphins[476,477,479] are powerful hormones controlling pain. Whereas, exorphins (e.g. morphine, Demerol, codeine, and heroin) require large doses (e.g. 10 mg morphine, 100 mg Demerol, etc), endorphins provide the same pain relief with 1/1000 smaller doses (e.g. 10–20 nanogram or billionth of gram). The similarities between endorphins and exorphins end at pain relief. Otherwise they act in a diametrically opposite fashion.

[b] Acid rain effect: alcohol as well as exorphins flood the brain cells and hamper their ability to form the dirunal hormones needed for alertness, sleep, tranquility, and antidepressant effects.

[c] Apparently the exorphins block the activation of adenylatecyclase, resulting in chronic tolerance.[566]

endorphins shows a similar location in the brain as well as quite a similar chemical structure of the polypeptides that form the three substances[92] (Figures 30 and 32).

ACTH is mainly an intermediary polypeptide. Its formation is stimulated by influences from neurotransmitters in the cortex and limbic system that induce the secretion of corticotropin-releasing factor (CRF) in the hypothalamus.

Via the portal venous system between the hypothalamus and pituitary, the CRF stimulates the formation of ACTH mainly in the pituitary gland.

Via the systemic circulation, ACTH induces the secretion of cortisol and other corticosteroids at the adrenal cortex.

This process is terminated by a negative feedback, i.e., cortisone formation inhibits the formation of ACTH, and ACTH formation inhibits the formation of CRF.

TRH AND CNS DEPRESSANTS

The corticopituitary end gland chain of events is not just limited to ACTH and CRF, but a similar system is present for thyroid-releasing hormone (TRH), thyroid-stimulating hormone (TSH), and thyroid hormone. Whereas TRH reverses the effect of barbiturates, alcohol,

TABLE 32
Endogenous Opioid Peptides

Endorphin: hexadecapeptide
        Rich concentration of opioid receptors
        Specific for the analgesic peptide
        Naloxone prevents immunochemical binding
        Caffeine has a similar effect
Enkephalin: pentapeptide
Dynorphin: mainly present in spinal cord and peripheral nerves, including sympathetic

benzodiazepines, and other sedatives, thus lessening the effects of the above-mentioned drugs, the thyroid hormone has the opposite effect. A similar system is also present for LH, luteinizing releasing hormone (LRH), and the eventual formation of estrogen.[29]

The final end organs are not just the adrenal gland, ovary, or thryoid gland; one vital final end organ is the gray matter of the brain stem. In this area, diurnal fluctuations of the above hormones result in diurnal changes of mood and alertness as well as morning wakefulness and evening drowsiness.

The negative feedback in the endocrine system (e.g., ACTH vs. CRF) plays a major role in the influence of polypeptides in different illnesses.

TABLE 33
Natural Endorphin Antagonists

β-endorphin 1–27
CCK (cholecystokinin)

The first step in management of chronic pain of RSD is to detoxify the patient from narcotics and benzodiazepines
    (BZ) so that the brain can form its own endorphins and benzodiazepines
The natural endorphin antagonists (Tables 36 and 37) stimulate further formation of endorphins. The exorphins
    (narcotics) do the opposite (Table 39)
Unfortunately the chronic pain of RSD is commonly treated with exorphins (narcotics) and exo-BZs (Table 41)
    (Xanax, valium, Halcion, etc.). Such chemicals perpetuate the pain and flood the CNS to the point that the brain
    becomes devoid of its own endorphins and BZs
Detoxification of each of the above two classes of medications is quite difficult. The combination of the two classes
    of addicting drugs (exorphins and BZs) makes the task several times more onerous and time-consuming. Quite
    frequently the patient is a closet drinker with the "acid rain" effect of alcohol further complicating the problem

HORMONES AND SEIZURE DISORDER

Since the 1950s it has been well recognized that corticolimbic hypothalamic hormones are usually anticonvulsants, whereas the end organ hormones lower the threshold for seizure disorder.

In infantile spasm (Lennox-Gastaut syndrome), administration of large doses of cortisone causes cerebral edema and a drop in the threshold of seizure and stimulates the formation of growth hormone by inhibiting the formation of CRF.

Secondarily the ACTH stimulation of growth hormone and TRH has a trophic effect on the immature and partially damaged cortex of the infantile spasm child. It not only controls the seizure disorder but improves the function as well as the potential growth of the cerebral hemispheres.

Prolactin raises the threshold for seizure and plays a major role in the termination of kindling effect of seizure. Pregnancy, sucking breast, TRH, insulin, and psychotropic drugs such as Tegretol increase the formation of prolactin and secondarily protect the brain against propagation of seizure activity.

On the other hand, norepinephrin, L-DOPA, ergotamines, and hypoglycemia lower the level of prolactin and lower the threshold for seizure disorder.

CLINICAL USES OF ACTH

ACTH is not an end-organ steroid such as cortisone or prednisone. In chronic pain patients as well as infants with cerebral damage, ACTH is far more comprehensive and effective in the management of the patients' medical problems than corticosteroids. It helps stimulate sex hormone, growth hormone, and endorphins, and by doing so, it has a multifactorial beneficial effect on RSD and chronic pain patients.

The dose is quite individualized, and we have noted that as little as 40 units i.m. once or twice a week or as much as 80 units i.m. two or three times a week can be quite effective in the treatment of such patients. The course of treatment should be limited to no more than 12 weeks, but the treatment can be repeated as closely as every 6 months.

ACTH IN TREATMENT OF PAIN AND RSD

ACTH and endorphins not only are structurally similar (Figure 30) they are found in similar structures in the brain. Their density fluctuates in a parallel fashion.

Endorphins are present at concentrations of 3 to 3.1 pg/ml in serums of normal individuals. ACTH is present in concentrations of 16 to 49 pg/ml.

In the central nervous system, ACTH and endorphins are found in similar sites.[412] The same peptides are present in stria terminalis, amygdaloid nuclei, and the fibers connecting the adjacent structures of limbic system to amygdaloid nuclei (Figure 21).

CSF endorphin levels drop in chronic pain or chronic use of narcotics. **Injection of insulin results in hypoglycemia and secondarily stimulates the formation of endorphins and ACTH.** As a result, during hypoglycemia the **serum endorphins rise** from 3 to 45 to 50 pmol/ml. A similar effect is noted in serum ACTH.[158]

The use of **exorphins** (narcotic abuse) **decreases the serum and CSF endorphins and ACTH.**

The use of **ACTH increases**[150] **the concentration of serum endorphins** from 3 to 38 pmol/ml.

The stimulation of endorphins secondarily results in **increase in prolactin, ACTH, growth hormone, and TSH.**

Reduction in endorphins or ACTH results in a reverse effect in regard to the above hormones, and results in a reduction in sex hormones.[14,207,412]

ACTH AND SEIZURE DISORDER

The effect on seizure disorder is quite similar for ACTH and endorphins. **ACTH, β-endorphins, CCK, and TRH are anticonvulsants**. On the other hand, **norepinephrin, vasopressin, and insulin,** as well as high doses of **corticosteroids, lower the threshold for seizure disorder**.[207]

ACTH is the anticonvulsant of choice in **infantile spasm** (**Lennox-Gastant** syndrome).

ACTH TREATMENT OF DEPRESSION IN RSD

Considerable research has sought to determine the focus of the hypothalamic-pituitary-adrenal axis abnormality in depression. The intracerebral ventricular adminstration of CRF in rats sets into motion behavioral and physiologic responses that are adaptive during threating situations. These responses include pituitary, adrenal, sympathetic, medullary activation, as well as arousal, anorexia, decreased libido, and hypothalamic hypogonadism.[357]

Severe depression usually results in markedly increased levels of cortisol in the blood at a magnitude at times resembling that seen in Cushing's disease.[114,150]

The following findings are proof that such a phenomenon is due to an increased CRF function.

1. Plasma ACTH responses to synthetic ovine CRF are attenuated in major depression, indicating that the **pituitary corticotropic hormone** is appropriately restrained by the negative biofeedback of cortisols.
2. Normal controls given a **continuous infusion of CRF** have the pattern and magnitude of hypercortisol levels in the blood seen in major depression.
3. CRF level of CSF is increased in patients affected by major depression. Cortisol responses to supraphysiological doses of ACTH (250 μg) have been reported to be elevated in depressed patients. In addition, in such severely depressed patients, post-mortem and CT studies have shown **enlarged adrenal gland** similar to **Cushing's disease**.[244] The use of **RU486**, which blocks cortisol receptors and produces increases in pituitary ACTH and greater endorphin secretion, demonstrates the biofeedback effect of increased ACTH activity in depressed patients.[244]
4. The frontal lobes cortex of suicide victims shows a marked reduction in corticosporin-releasing binding sites as compared to controls.[244]

Depression manifests itself in two opposite forms:

1. A tendency for eating, hypertension, and poor sleep such as seen with Cushing's disease.
2. Anorexia, hypotension, anxiety, and insomnia.

In the first group, the use of ACTH aggravates the depression, whereas in the second group, our present research studies are revealing strong beneficial effects of ACTH in treatment of **anorexia nervosa** (study in progress).

Anorexia nervosa has been reported to be associated with RSD.[338] In our experience, both anorexia and RSD respond positively to treatment with ACTH.

These two conditions are nothing but a manifestation of the complex biofeedback endocrine system in neuropsychiatric illnesses.

Recent studies are developing standard laboratory tests that measure plasma ACTH, cortisol, and β-endorphins before and after 1 μg/kg of ovine CRF. These studies reveal the parallel increase in the concentration of ACTH, β-endorphins, and cortisol in plasma of normal individuals.

However, with higher doses of CRF cortisol levels stay high, but the ACTH and endorphin levels drop.[244] This may explain the depressing effect of long-term use of corticosteroids and the opposite effect of ACTH.

ESTROGENS (also see TRH and CNS Depressants)

Menopausal drop of serum estrogen as well as reduction of serum estrogen by alcohol and cigarettes aggravates RSD, with further surface vasoconstriction, deep bone wash-out osteoporosis, and perpetuation of pain. Correction of the above factors is essential in treatment of chronic pain and RSD. Even prior to menopause, the above drug abuses (ETOH and cigarettes) cause spondylosis which is erroneously and most frequently is mistaken for "arthritis". Nonsteroidal analgesic drugs (NSAD) are used with no benefit. Estrogen therapy is quite helpful in female osteoporosis,[480] and in RSD.

ANTIDEPRESSANTS

Antidepressants are analgesic[17] and are the treatment of choice for chronic pain. RSD is an exaggerated form of chronic pain, so it is obvious that antidepressants would be the treatment of choice for RSD.

Amitriptyline exaggerates and augments morphine analgesia due to its direct effect on CNS.[34] Of the two groups of antidepressants, the ones that enhance the accumulation of norepinephrine at synapses obviously would have a deleterious effect on management of RSD. The preferred form of treatment is the antidepressants which increase the serotonin concentration of synapse or at least are more likely to increase extracellular serotonin than norepinephrine concentration.

Antidepressants, through blockage of serotonin receptors in CNS, activate **descending pain inhibitory fibers** in the brain stem and result in analgesia.

Trazodone[231,238,239,321] is quite effective and well tolerated. It helps control chronic pain and also provides an antidepressant and sedative effect. It does not cause the hypotensive and cardiac side effects of tricyclic antidepressants.

Tricyclic antidepressants, especially desipramine, are quite palliative and may be curative[110] in diabetic neuropathy. These painful conditions are best treated with antidepressants and nerve block.

Tricyclic antidepressants potentiate and accentuate the effect of morphine analgesia.[17] The application of tricyclics that can cause orthostatic hypotension (e.g., amitriptyline) should be discouraged in RSD patients.

MANAGEMENT OF INSOMNIA

Insomnia is an integral part of the complex chronic pain (CCP) RSD. "The pain that never stops" does not relent at night. CCP deprives the patient of rapid eye movement (REM) sleep. This in turn results in disruption of cerebral function the next day. This electrochemical cerebral dysfunction results in frustration, agitation, and fatigue, i.e., depression.

The management of CCP-induced insomnia and secondary depression should be achieved by the following:

1. Avoidance of the application and replacement of endogenous hormones and chemicals such as benzodiazepines and narcotics.
2. A comprehensive diet, exercise, and antidepressant treatment.

Insomnias are classified as

1. Transient insomnia, e.g., jet lag or acute distress.
2. Short-term insomnia (adjustment dyssomnia), e.g., family or job loss distress.
3. Long-term insomnia.

Long-term insomnia is in turn subdivided into

1. Early evening insomnia, e.g., acute or subacute distress, drug effect (coffee).
2. Early morning arousal, e.g., time zone change; more commonly insomnia due to presenile or senile dementia.
3. Interrupted sleep, e.g., depression. This class is the most common group of insomnias encountered by algologists and neurologists.

The treatment of choice for Class 3 (interrupted sleep) typical of CCP of RSD is

1. Diet: Food rich in serotoninergic tryptophan (dairy products and fruits) and low in tyrosine (red meat, red wine) are to be consumed at night (Table 22).
2. Antidepressants, especially trazodone, which increases REM sleep frequency without systemic side effects.

TABLE 34
Ephaptic and Epileptogenic Scars

Fibrous tissue with low electrolyte exchange
Decreased capillaries
Denudation
Deafferentation hypersensitivity
Decreased inhibitory cells and dendrites in CNS scars

BZ Hypnotics
1. Flurazepam (Dalmane): half-life, 8 hours; N, desalkyl, Flurazepam (NDF) — its metabolite — half-life 50-300 hours causes depression, poor memory, daytime sedation
2. Temazepam (Restoril): half-life, 8 hours: side effects — poor memory, depression
3. Triazolam (Halcion™): a dangerous hypnotic: half-life 5 hours; longer metabolite binding effect
    a. Strong receptor binding to brain stem (BZ1): strongly addictive
    b. Strong receptor binding to hippocampus (BZ2): confusion, poor memory, depression, anxiety
    c. Withdrawal: daytime anxiety even with occasional use

Insomnia
1. Acute anxiety type: insomnia at onset of sleep
    Rx: L-tryptophane in dairy products; avoidance of ETOH; Rx with chloral hydrate
2. Chronic, intractable anxiety (CIA) with resultant depression: disrupted sleep with frequent awakening
    Rx: antidepressants, e.g., Trazodone (50–100 mg); avoidance of ETOH
3. Cerebral atrophy: early morning awakening
    Aging: usually no Rx needed
    Alcoholism: abstinence, chloral hydrate
    Advanced atrophy: Thioridazine (Mellaril)
                        Haloperidol

Endogenous Benzodiazepines (ENDO-BZ)
1. Endo-diazepam: 3 pmol/cc in CSF
    a. In ETOH hepatic encephalopathy the CSF endo-diazepam is 30 pmol/cc (10x normal)
    b. Flumozemil, diazepam antagonist, rapidly reverses hepatic encepahlopthy
    c. Nonhepatic encephalopathic patients have normal CSF endo-diazepam (J. Rothstein, et al., *Ann. Neurol.*, 1990)
2. N-desmethyldiazepam, and 4 other diazepam metabolites, potentiate GABA activity of cerebral cortex

FIGURE 33. Benzodiazepine (BZ) binding to the receptors in the brain and insomnia and BZ.

None of these measures will do any good if the standard hypnotics of benzodiazepine or barbiturate families are used, or if the patient consumes alcohol (which deprives the patient of REM sleep) or narcotics (patient wakes up every 3 hours for next fix of narcotics).

Simply put, the cause of insomnia (depression) should be addressed to achieve proper sleep.

The universal method of shutting the patient up with strong benzodiazepines (BZ) is apt to deteriorate the pain and depression as well as compounding the disease by another disease — addiction — and increasing the risk of suicide (see Table 34 and Figure 33).

ANTICONVULSANTS

In certain forms of severe RSD (i.e., major causalgias, postherpetic RSD, and RSD due to electrical injury) due to electric short ephapse, a severe electric shock type of pain develops in the periphery, and **myoclonic** and **akinetic seizures** occur if the scar is in the spinal cord or brain stem (Table 34).

TABLE 35
Tendency for Benzodiazepine Binding in Diencephalic — Limbic System[a]

Most binding[b] (dependence)	Average days (detox)	Medium binding	Average days	Least binding[c]	Average days
Triazolam	68	Alprazolam	8	Clonazepam	2
Lorazepam	27			Oxazepam	3
Diazepam	25				
Clorzepate	23				
Chlordiazepoxide	12				

[a] A study of 316 patients detoxified at Neurological Associates, Vero Beach and New Horizons, Ft. Pierce, FL.
[b] The most binding group has the highest tendency to dependence, and a few weeks of detoxification is not enough.
[c] The least binding group (Clonazepam and Oxazepam) did not need detoxification. They were additional drugs among prescription narcotics group that required admission.

In such cases, anticonvulsants may render a significant relief.[60,81,205,283,365] Tegretol[7] (but not the generic carbamazepine) and Clonazepam are far more effective than Phenytoin.

Even though Clonazepam is a BZ, and hence a depressant, it has a very low affinity to BZ receptors. It usually is nonaddictive and is an effective anticonvulsant.

Anticonvulsants suppress pathological electrical (ectopic) discharges both in the CNS and peripheral nervous system.[7,365,373] To a lesser extent, Phenytoin and valporic acid may be helpful.[283,365]

ANTIVIRAL TREATMENT

Postherpetic neuralgia is a model of RSD in its manifestations and management.

Early diagnosis is essential. The common eruptive form is easy to diagnose. The uncommon noneruptive form can easily be diagnosed in early Stage I with the help of thermography.

Early treatment with a combination of acylovir (800 mg tid or qid), dexamethasone, or prednisone, as well as topical application of Capsaicin® is very effective. If treatment is delayed over 3 to 6 months, it is apt to fail.

DISCONTINUATION OF NARCOTICS AND BENZODIAZEPINES

Narcotics and benzodiazepines (BZ) lock into the corresponding receptor sites in brain stem. Three to four hours later withdrawal causes repetitive use. The brain stops making its own endorphins and BZs. As a result, pain and depression become exaggerated.

Usually ephaptic dystrophies are accompanied by such multiple pain factors that they require multiple discipline therapies and a flexible understanding and empathy on the part of the treating physician. Some of these patients become worse with heat application and some become worse with change of temperature. They are invariably accompanied by severe anxiety and depression.

The use of benzodiazepines, narcotics, and alcohol in such patients should be avoided. Either in the form of sleeping pills or tranquilizers, **benzodiazepines invariably aggravate central pain** by depleting endogenous diazepines in the brain stem and limbic system.

As benzodiazepines bind the BZ receptors in the brain stem and limbic system ("lock and key phenomenon"), they reduce the cerebral generation of ENDO-BZs with resultant drug dependence (Table 35, Figure 33). The following BZs have the least tendency for binding — hence, less dependence: (1) clonazepam and (2) oxazepam.

Buspiron and thioridazine (Mellaril) are less problematic than BZs in chronic pain and RSD patients.

BIOFEEDBACK (OPERANT CONDITIONING)

Ever since the seminal work of Pavlov at the turn of this century followed by Skinner's contributions a few decades later, brain power has been utilized for positive and negative operant conditioning.

Conditioning the brain through Nauta's SHMLC (septohypothalamo-mesencephalic-limbic complex) controls both conscious and autonomic cerebral function (Figure 21b).

Shearn[485] showed the power of conditioned reflex (operant conditioning) to change human heart rate. As is the case with all operant conditioning reflexes, proper reward that stimulates hypothalamic and brain stem pleasure centers enables the animal to achieve somatic as well as autonomic manipulation of function (Trowill[486]). Dicara and Miller[486] trained the animal to vasodilate the dermal vessels in one ear and to constrict the arterial flow in the opposite ear.

Biofeedback — teaching subjects what they are expected to do — has been proven to be an effective therapeutic tool since original works of Brever in 1962.[487] Biofeedback, combined with yoga[488] or transcendental meditation,[489] can reduce hypertension by 20 mm Hg, and may prevent the need for surgical treatment for arterial occlusion.[490]

Biofeedback is quite effective for treatment of headache, both by achieving muscle relaxation and by achieving vasodilation (Appenzeller[489]).

Biofeedback is an accessory and complementary treatment. It is one step closer to distress avoidance: diet, exercise, relaxation, meditation, etc. It is not considered curative for a severe disease such as RSD, but in this disease a multidisciplinary approach is the key to the control of pain.

Treatment with a combination of **Baclofen**, **sympathetic block**, and physiotherapy is quite effective for spasticity and flexion deformity of RSD. In advanced cases, treatment with **botulism toxin** (**Botox**®) injection of neuromuscular junctions is quite effective.

INVASIVE NERVE BLOCKS

SYMPATHETIC GANGLION NERVE BLOCKS

Early diagnosis, physiotherapy, and sympathetic ganglia nerve block are essential in management of RSD.

Local anesthetics are used both for diagnostic and therapeutic purposes. Mepivacaine (0.5%) and bupivacaine (0.25%) are usually used with a duration of 1–3 and 3–4 hours, respectively.[269]

The nerve block is done on accessible areas such as the stellate ganglion nerve block for head and upper extremities and lumbar sympathetic ganglion nerve block for lower extremities. Celiac ganglion nerve block is also done quite frequently for abdominal manifestations of RSD. The block is done for both diagnostic and therapeutic purposes.

The nerve block is best done in the hands of an experienced anesthesiologist. An anesthesiologist who has a subspecialty in performing nerve blocks can help **reduce mortality** and morbidity.

In cases of stellate ganglion nerve block, which is quite effective in the management of RSD, lack of experience or expertise can expose the patient to side effects such as death due to inadvertant injection into the vertebral artery.[199,227]

For effective treatment of chronic RSD, **repetitive nerve blocks** are frequently necessary. The repeated nerve blocks are very effective in the successful cure of RSD when combined with physiotherapy. However, repetitive nerve blocks also increase the chances of mortality and morbidity if not done by an expert.

Bier block (regional block) is the blockade of choice when repetitive blocks are needed for RSD of the upper extremity. **Repetitive stellate blocks** are dangerous and should be avoided.

Nerve blocks are very helpful in diabetic neuropathy RSD as well as traumatic RSD.

Sympathetic Block for Efferent Complications of RSD

Nerve block is not only effective in control of pain and inactivity in RSD, but also is very effective in the cure of efferent motor side effects of RSD. These consist of dystonias, tremors of different types, flexion deformities, extension of the knees, flexion of the elbows and wrists, and even motor (paresis) secondary to chronic RSD. Sympathetic nerve block under these conditions is quite effective and curative[127,425] (Table 37).

The efferent dystonic and paresthetic dysfunction secondary to RSD is recognized in clinical practice[127,326,425] and in laboratory animals in experiments with sympathetic stimulators and blockers, which have demonstrated a disturbance of motor function both in regard to muscle contraction as well as inactivity and weakness.[45,119,132,145,179,259,260,371,404,405,414,420]

Sympathetic Ganglion Block and Motor Dysfunction of RSD: Hemifacial Spasm and Blepharospasm

Neilsen[245–247] reported hemifacial spasm due to ephaptic nerve damage.

In our study of RSD manifestations, three patients had blepharospasm due to facial RSD after injury to the ophthalmic (trigeminal) nerve.

All three patients had total relief with stellate ganglion block. A fourth patient with blepharospasm suffered from cervical spondylosis (Figure 23 and Table 13) and a combination of articular facet injection in the cervical spinal muscles at the C4–5 level on the right side and stellate ganglion block cured her blepharospasm.

Dystonia

The sympathetic ganglion block is curative for dystonia and flexion deformities, and corrects muscle atrophy in the extremity when combined with physiotherapy.

Yokota et al.[425] as well as Schwartzman[332] reported on patients who were partially

TABLE 36
Complications of Stellate Sympathetic Block

Horner's syndrome (temporary — a sign of effective block)
Pneumothorax (extremely rare)
Bradycardia (right stellate block)
Vertebral artery injection (seizure; even death)
Brachial plexus block (indicates needle is anterior to C6 vertebra)
Inability to cough (hoarse voice, recurrent laryngeal nerve injection)
Epidural or subdural injection

TABLE 37
Complications of Lumbar Sympathetic Block

Perforation of disc
Somatic nerve damage, e.g., genitourinary nerve damage or sciatic damage
Vertebral structures damage
Vena cava or aortic perforation
Kidney damage
Orthostatic hypotension in bilateral blocks
In rare cases aberrant manifestation of RSD seen
    Horner's syndrome
    RSD in the hand in a patient with no previous
    RSD in upper extremities

paralyzed or had marked weakness of the extremities secondary to RSD and treated with sympathetic block.

They demonstrated loading of epinephrine, norepinephrine, and isoproterenol injections decreased the muscle strength of the affected limb in such patients. On the other hand, loading injections of pilocarpine, atropine, or edrophonium did not influence the strength of the muscles.

REGIONAL BLOCK

Regional i.v. infusion of reserpine or stellate ganglion block improved the strength of the muscles in the involved extremities. This improvement was quite dramatic in all patients. On the other hand, placebo loading had no effect on muscle strength.

Yokota et al.[425] reported improvement of ptosis by the sympathetic ganglion block in spite of the development of Horner's syndrome. They explained that the improvement of ptosis is due to the improvement of muscle strength of the right frontal and levator palpebrae muscles. They also showed that i.v. administration of reserpine or propranolol resulted in improvement of bilateral ptosis.

FATIGUE AND SYMPATHETIC NERVE BLOCK: ORBELI PHENOMENON

Orbeli[259] reported an antifatigue action by the sympathetic nervous system on skeletal muscles (Orbeli effect).[259,371] In rabbits, repetitive stimulation of sympathetic ganglion can result in paralysis of the hind legs.[414]

Yokota et al.[425] referred to the above phenomenon of muscle weakness in the extremities due to sympathetic dystrophy as "sympathetic motor paresis". It is obvious that sympathetic motor paresis is only one of the many manifestations of efferent motor dysfunction of the muscles in the extremities secondary to RSD.

REPETITIVE SYMPATHETIC NERVE BLOCK FOR
MANIFESTATIONS OF RSD

The sympathetic nerve block should be initiated promptly. Prompt blockage, early diagnosis, and aggressive physiotherapy are the key factors in successful management of RSD.[224,244a,308]

The type of nerve block is dictated by first, what the patient can tolerate, and second, how early the disease has been diagnosed. For early stages of RSD, cervical or lumbar sympathetic block with local anesthetic agents is quite successful and the treatment of choice. The more chronic the illness, the more repetitive nerve blocks are necessary.

In the earliest stages of RSD, one to four blocks may be all the patient needs.

In the more advanced stages of RSD, usually the patient needs a series of blocks. As the blocks are repeated, the patient gets longer lasting relief after each block.

In advanced cases, after several blocks, the patient may need nerve blocks only once every 9 months to a year.

REGIONAL BLOCKS

Early diagnosis, early block, and the teamwork of neurologist, physiatrist, and anesthesiologist are required for successful results of treatment.

Regional pharmacologic block is a universally considered effective and frequently used mode of therapy. The specific technique varies; however, it usually consists of infiltration of a long-acting anesthetic agent, such as bupivacaine hydrochloride, in the region of the lumbar sympathetic chain. If administered early in the course of the syndrome, persistent pain relief may be obtained from a single block. However, usually blocks must be repeated daily or every other day until pain is controlled. It can be diagnostic as well: if the patient's pain is due to conversion reaction (17% of chronic pain patients) injection of normal saline causes good relief.[478]

Stellate ganglion block can cause serious complications. The complications are magnified when, as is usally the case, repetitive blocks are required. In such patients, regional block is a better alternative.

Bier block[28] with guanethidine or reserpine is indicated when ganglion nerve blocks cannot be done.

Technically, the extremity is isolated from general circultation by a 30–100 Torr above systolic blood pressure. Reserpine (1–2 mg) or guanethidine (10–20 mg) is then applied.

In patients who are under anticoagulation treatment or are allergic to anesthetic medications, regional i.v. with guanethidine or reserpine[126–128,243] may be quite effective.

Bier block[28] avoids side effects such as pneumothorax, intradural, or extradural injection, Horner's syndrome, anhydrosis, and death due to injection into the vertebral artery. Its effect also may last longer than the ganglion block. However, it is somewhat painful. In experienced hands of Hannington-Kiff[126–128] up to 80% relief of pain can be achieved for over 15 weeks. He emphasized that regional block is preferred to ganglionic block and usually is the only block needed for complete relief.[421]

Guanethidine causes expulsion of norepinephrine at the nerve ending. The half-life of guanethidine is quite prolonged. A single injection of guanethidine has a 50% excretion rate of 2 to 3 days through the kidneys.[248] The duration of regional block with guanethidine has been reported from days up to months.[12,48,74,127,128,144,200,253]

Regional block should be immediately followed by physiotherapy. Simple block without physiotherapy has far higher failure rate.

Early diagnosis, early block, and the teamwork of physiatrist and anesthesiologist are required for successful results of treatment.

The use of regional corticosteroids during regional blocks enhances mobilization of joints and helps relieve chronic pain.

METHOD

The method reported by Poplawski is in common use.[280] It should be done by an anesthesiologist. After insertion of a small needle into a vein on the dorsum of the extremity, the limb is exsanguinated by elevating it for 2 minutes and a pneumatic tourniquet is inflated to higher than systolic blood pressure. For an upper extremity, the tourniquet is applied to below the shoulder at a pressure of 250 to 300 mm Hg. For a lower extremity, the pressure is applied around the calf at 300 to 350 mm Hg. A mixture of 25–30 ml of 1% xylocaine (without epinephrine) and 80 mg of Solu-Medrol is injected into the vein.

The block generally lasts up to 30 minutes. Manipulation procedures are done. During the block, Brand and Curtis' method of manipulation is applied.[46] Manipulation and massage are combined. After 30 minutes, the tourniquet is reclosed for 30 seconds. This is repeated two to three times before termination of the block. Each block is followed by extensive physiotherapy.

Poplawski[280] reports a 75% success rate with this block.

Multidisciplinary treatment combined with sympathetic blockage or regional blockage is necessary for successful management of RSD.

This multidisciplinary treatment consists of physiotherapy, antidepressants for treatment of chronic pain, trigger point injections, TNS, oral sympatholytic medications, or at times calcium channel blockers.

These treatments spare the patient from other invasive and unsuccessful treatments. Other invasive treatments such as sympathectomy, epidural dorsal column stimulators, and thalamic stimulation result in excellent short-term benefits and disastrous long-term effects. The plain combination of aggressive physiotherapy and regional block and sympathetic block has been reported to be effective and successful in up to 80% of patients.[37,398] The effect of nerve block in the case of ephaptic RSD is quite variable and it is not at all unusual for the patient to notice aggravation of the burning pain after nerve block. This temporary aggravation is not in the form of aggravation of reticular pain, but it is an allodynia and quite an unpleasant burning pain focalized to the area of ephaptic nerve damage and dysfunction.

In this regard, the block can be diagnostic to localize the origin of the ephaptic nerve damage. This is not exactly as diagnostic as thermography would be, but it is a good adjunct diagnostic tool.

Repetitive ganglion blocks usually take away the temporary aggravation of the pain and should not discourage the therapist from repeating the injections.

INVASIVE TREATMENT

Except for the use of a morphine pump in rare selective cases, invasive treatment is useless in RSD. Long term, sympathectomy, tractotomy, rhizotomy, as well as invasive spinal cord stimulation are apt to fail. Even short term, amputation of extremity (for treatment of multiple Sudek's atrophy fractures) is apt to fail. By and large, if they help the patient on a long-term basis, the patient is getting nothing but a placebo effect. Hence, the treatment would not have been necessary to begin with.

Palliative surgery may make sense for patients who are not expected to live long (e.g., due to advanced diabetic complications). In such patients with short life expectancy, sympathectomy makes sense as it provides relief for less than 5 years.

SYMPATHECTOMY

Sympathectomy is very helpful in the first 2- to 5-year postoperative period. If the patient has a short life expectancy due to diabetes or hypertension, then it is logical to proceed with this operation.

Sympathectomy was first performed by Leriche[189] in 1916. Since then, after each major war, sympathectomy has been a popular treatment of RSD. During each war and immediately after the war, glorious results have been obtained by sympathectomy. These have been due to the fact that the patients have been referred to surgeons for urgent relief. The patients who have

TABLE 38
Regional Block

Advantages
    Avoids pneumothorax
    Avoids Horner's syndrome
    Avoids inadvertant extra or individual injection
    Avoids death due to vertebral artery injection
Disadvantages
    Painful
    Needs a lot of experience
Complications
    Transient vertigo and tinnitus
    Transient numbness and carpopedal spasms in extremities
    Superficial infection
    Superficial thrombophlebitis

Regional block as well as ganglion block without aggressive physiotherapy are doomed to fail
Epidural block
    Epidural block with combination of corticosteroids and anesthetics is a very helpful adjunct to physiotherapy

had good results have been the ones who have responded satisfactorily to diagnostic sympathetic blocks.[38] It is not clear if the same patients could have had just as good results with repetitive blocks.[136]

TECHNIQUE

Surgical textbooks review the technique in detail. This is an update in the review by Bonica.[456]

Sympathectomy is achieved by three methods:

1.   Neurolytic block: up to 10T phenol or up to 100% alcohol injected in contrast medium
2.   Radiofrequency lesions
3.   Surgical sympathectomy

The neurolytic block should be strongly discouraged because of its target inaccuracy and more importantly because the phenol or alcohol leaves new scars and new sources of pain.

The radiofrequency method in the hands of Wilkinson[416,417] has resulted in some improvement in sympathetic pain. As with other methods, it has not been impressively helpful in management of causalgia.[457,458]

Surgical approaches are time-honored since Leriche[189] with few variations in technique.

Upper thoracic sympathectomy is achieved by a posterior paravertebral approach, auxillary transthoracic approach, or supraclavicular (retropleural) method.[416,417] The rate of development of Horner's syndrome is variable depending on which method is used.[459,460]

Lumbar sympathectomy[459] is achieved through a posterior paravertebral approach or anterior oblique method.

RESULTS

There has been no definitive long-term study to assess the exact rate of success after surgical sympathectomy. Tables 39a, 39b, and Figure 35 summarize our experience with long-term follow-up of 48 patients after sympathectomy. These patients were followed as a part of chronic pain evaluation, and they were followed from 15 to 19 years.

Successful responses to sympathectomy have been reported in the literature in 12 to 97% of patients.[389,413] There are two reasons for such a discrepancy: first is the difference between short-term vs. long-term follow-up of the patients. The longer patients are followed after

TABLE 39a
Sympathectomy in Peacetime RSD[a]

Excellent (no pain)	Good (75% relief)	Fair (25% relief)	Failure
2 (4.2%)	28 (58.3%)	2 (4.2%)	18 (33.3%)
0	19 (39.5%)	6 (12.5%)	23 (48%)
0	5 (10%)	4* (8.3%)	39 (81.25%)

Forty-eight patients, 15 years follow-up.

TABLE 39b
Sympathectomy in Wartime Causalgia[a]

War	Results		
	Excellent	Fair	No relief
WWII, French Colonial War, Vietnam War, 518 operations	83%	12%	5%

Summary of results from Bonica.[38]

sympathectomy, the higher the rate of failure. Secondly, wartime sympathectomies followed by return of the soldiers. This emotional reward after sympathectomy has a potent and positive therapeutic effect. The same doesn't apply to peacetime sympathectomy patients.

In addition, sympathectomy can cause postsympathectomy pain called **sympathalgia** in up to 44% of patients undergoing this procedure.[375,389] This is usually seen after lumbar sympathectomy, and development of such a complication is higher after chemical than after surgical sympathectomy.

The sympathalgia secondary to sympathectomy usually starts around the first 2 weeks of the surgical procedure. It is a dull and cramping pain and occasionally can be a sharp pain.[286] Although it is temporary in some patients, in other patients it can persist for several months or years.

Experience with chronic pain patients in pain clinics away from the theatre of a war does not show such satisfactory results from sympathectomy.

The present trend goes along with the repetitive cautious stance of Sunderland.[363]

Sympathectomy usually causes practically 100% relief in the first few months; and after 2 to 7 years, the rate of success drops to 15 to 30% (Tables 39 and 40 and Figure 35); a placebo effect alone produces around 17% success. Success up to 3 months to less than a year after surgery is very impressive and has been reported in up to 88–100% of patients.[35,37,398] However, long-term (up to 10 years or over) follow-up shows a failure rate of over 71% in 36 consecutive patients.[37,398] Forty-eight patients followed by us over 15 years show a low success rate after sympathectomy for RSD (Tables 39a and 39b).

CAUSES OF FAILURE AFTER SYMPATHECTOMY

1. Sympathectomy is analogous to the act of killing the messenger. The sympathetic nervous system has the critical job of properly controlling and preserving the circulation in different parts of the body, especially in the extremities. By paralyzing the system, the extremity will be more apt to have disturbance of circulation and is left unprotected from fluctuations in circulation.

Sympathectomy is similar to permanently removing the central heat and air-conditioning system and never replacing it because of malfunction.

TABLE 40
Factors Contributing to Sympathectomy Failure

Sympathetic nervous system is bilaterally and symmetrically innervated. Unilateral sympathectomy cannot be
  complete
Bilateral sympathetctomy has too many side effects (e.g., hypotension, impotence)
SNS is anatomically primitive and structurally inconsistent.[479a] Amoebic-type connections of the ganglia makes "total
  sympathetctomy" impossible (Figure 34)
Overlapping SNS thermatomal innervation results in postsympathectomy regeneration
Cannon's phenomenon (topical noradrenergic autonomy) at the area of ephapse perpetuates the postsympathectomy
  pain
Spread of RSD to adjacent structures results in new manifestations of RSD in remote arease, e.g., Horner's syndrome
  or de novo RSD of hand after lumbar sympathectomy
The permanent destruction of thermoregulatory function of SNS causes latent complications, e.g., RSD in contralat-
  eral extremity
War and peace RSD and war and peace medical (e.g., dibenzyline treatment resuls in Lebanese war)[62] and surgical
  results are not identical and comparable (see Tables 39 and 42)
The war casualties are more likely to be stress-induced analgesia (SIA) than peacetime trauma (e.g., a work injury
  is more likely to be stress-induced pain — SIP — because of legal complications). SIA pain responds better to
  treatment
Repeated sympathectomies are invariably doomed to fail[36]

Sympathectomy permanently damages the temperature regulatory system. The reason sympathectomy does not cause side effects other than ineffective control of pain as well as impotence and orthostatic hypotension is because it is invariably partial and incomplete.

2. Even after "complete" removal of the sympathetic plexus for the upper or lower extremities, the sympathetic nerves in the wall of blood vessels are left intact.

3. As shown in Table 6, the most common form (over 80%) of RSD is disuse RSD. In this situation, the sympathetic system is temporarily hyperactive. Proper conservative treatment would prevent any unnecessary invasive surgery (such as sympathectomy) in such patients.

4. Usually the patients that end up needing sympathectomy are the ones who suffer from **ephaptic dystrophy**. Sympathectomy in such cases causes a classic **Cannon phenomenon** (Figure 7). This physiological phenomenon refers to the fact that the end organ that is controlled by sympathetic nerve fibers will become uninhibited in its chemical dysfunction. As a result, even though the sympathetic fibers are not contributing to acetylcholine or norepinephrine secretion at the area of nerve damage, the partially damaged sensory nerves become uninhibited with resultant increase of pain input.

In diabetic neuropathy RSD,[477a] sympathetctomy dramatically relieves the pain for the first 1 to 3 years. Then deafferentation and Cannon phenomenon set in. As a result, invariably by the second to fifth year the patient ends up with a lot more pain. Sympathetic blocks repeated every 6 to 12 months yield similar results.

In patients who have had sympathectomy, thermography shows an increase of temperature in the focus of ephaptic nerve damage (Cannon phenomenon) with secondary increase of pain and discomfort (Figure 7).

5. There is a significant overlap in the border areas of sympathetic nerve dermatomes. As a result, the adjacent intact sympathetic nerves try to overcome the lack of sympathetic input. This contributes to the failure of long-term effects of symptathectomy.

6. Whereas the neospinothalamic tract is quite consistent in its anatomical pattern, the sympathetic nerves and plexi are phylogenetically old, and show a marked individual variability in humans. This causes a problem at the time of surgery and results in the gray rami branching off and entering in a few adjacent areas of the sympathetic paravertebral chain. As a result, the removal of part of this chain does not guarantee a "complete" sympathectomy.

7. The sympathetic nervous system functions symmetrically and bilaterally[176,332] (Figure 34). So the removal of a portion of this system on one side does not achieve a "total" sympathectomy.

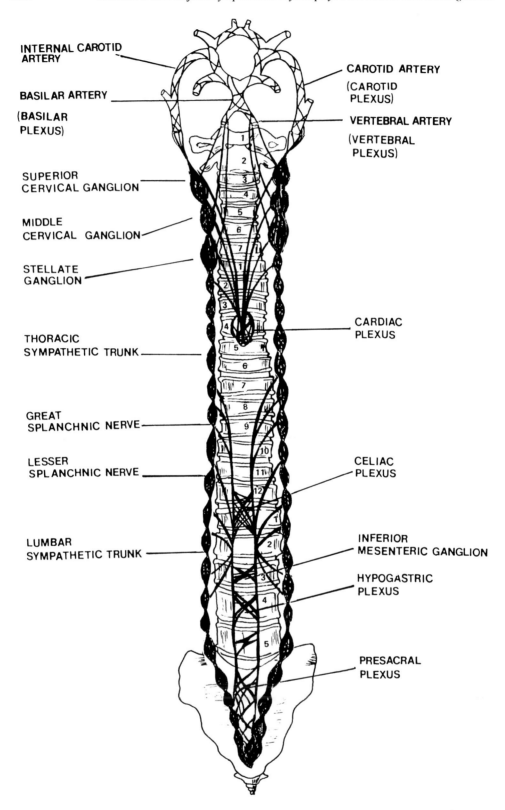

FIGURE 34. Vertical and midline connections and plexi of SNS. This complex intermingling of the SNS fibers renders unilateral sympathectomy ineffective in the long run.

Sympathectomy in Wartime Causalgia
518 Patients

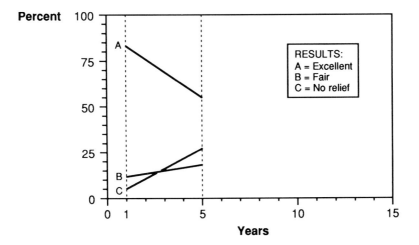

Sympathectomy in Peacetime RSD
48 Patients
(1971-1990)

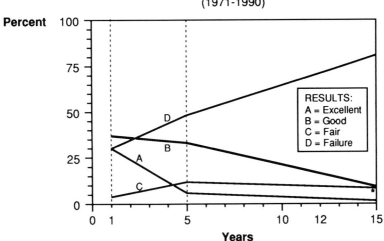

* 2 patients required morphine pump, 1 patient required ECT

FIGURE 35. Failure of sympathectomy after 5 years or longer follow-up.

8. At times when patients undergo lumbar sympathectomy, we have noted that they may develop Horner's syndrome on the same side or marked vasoconstriction of the hand on the same side, reflecting the complex and primitive connections of the sympathetic nervous system. Cooper[483a] has shown vasoconstriction in the hand during electrical stimulation of the lumbar sympathetic chain. We have noted development of *de novo* RSD in the ipsilateral hand in two patients after lumbar sympathetic block.

9. Repeated sympathectomies are no guarantee of success.[19]

TABLE 41
War and Peace Causalgias

War causalgia	Peace causalgias[a]
90% of battlefield causalgias are above elbow and knee[461]	80% of causalgias in our series of 101 patients with RSD involve dorsum of foot and below elbow regions

A study of 101 RSD patients followed over 5 years

RSD of disuse	82
Ephaptic RSD[a]	19
	Total 101

Minor causalgias		11
Brachial plexus injury	(1)	
Contusion	(1)	
Injury dorsum of foot	(1)	
Injury forearm or hand	(4)	
Major causalgias		8
Injury dorsum of foot	(5)	
Injury forearm or hand	(3)	
		Total 19

[a] Below knee or elbow 16/19 (80%).

10. Another side effect of sympathectomy is that the patient loses motivation for physiotherapy and exercise. Because sympathectomy results in immediate relief in the first few months, the patient has less inclination or motivation to exercise and help improve the circulation of the extremity.

11. Even in the cases of rare and severe major causalgias, it makes more sense to resort to a morphine pump than to sympathectomy (Table 42).

The application of sympathectomy in management of RSD should be strongly discouraged.

If the patient suffering from RSD has a short life expectancy (less than 5 years), then sympathectomy makes sense and should be done.

MORPHINE PUMP

After all fails, resort to Morphine pump which provides nice relief of pain.

If all fails in advanced stage 3 and 4 RSD, a Morphine pump[567–572] provides very good relief and avoids self-medication by the patient. Patients entrusted with the use of narcotics for chronic pain are caught in the vicious circle of replacing endorphins with exorphins in an accelerating fashion. This means the pain wakes the patient up every 2–3 hours due to the rapid drop in serum level of exorphines. As a result, REM sleep is aborted, depression is aggravated, and pain threshold is reduced.

The morphine pump, and for that matter the sulfentanil (fentanyl)[569,570] pump (a synthetic narcotic 100 times stronger than morphine) infuses in the CSF several times less of a narcotic dose than does an oral or i.m. form of narcotic administration.

The application of a morphine pump provides a steady-state and smaller dose of morphine and excludes volitional self-administration by the patient. In a dozen of our patients suffering from RSD, a morphine pump has provided total pain relief. Its main complication of respiratory depression is dose-related.

The physician should be quite discriminative in selecting patients for this procedure. An objective neuropsychometric test is essential. This will help identify patients who have high scores for an hysterical profile and who are more likely to have persistent pain afterward. A high score for depression is common among RSD patients and is no contraindication for further treatment. The depression usually improves with better control of pain. Miller and Dekatas[226] found no difference in psychological profiles of RSD patients compared with other patients. However, in chronic pain of any form, there is a tendency for secondary gain (conversion reaction) in one sixth of these patients (Table 7). Such patients respond poorly to any form of treatment.

PATIENT-CONTROLLED ANALGESIA (PCA)

This computerized method of morphine (or fentanyl) pump allows the patient to self-administer narcotics.

This method should be limited to the final stages of advanced cancer, and to bone transplant patients suffering from cancer. It is definitely contraindicated in chronic pain — especially RSD — patients.

In our study of eight RSD patients treated with a morphine pump and followed for over 24 months, there was no tendency for increased demand of analgesic. (The other four — done in the past 2 years — have not needed any more pain medication.)

This is in contrast to advanced cancer patients who require increasing doses of analgesic because their pain is not a chronic pain, but is an acutely progressive and destructive pain.

Similar beneficial results have been observed in patients suffering from other noncancerous chronic pain such as nerve roots contusion, arachnoiditis, and Landry-Guillian-Barré syndrome.

In some cancer patients with severe intractable pain, a combination of fentanyl and morphine has been applied intrathecally. This treatment is frought with respiratory depression and should not be used for intractable chronic pain such as seen in RSD patients.

Combined application of a morphine pump and oral carbamazepine (Tegretol, not generic) helps some cancer patients. There is, however, no such reports in RSD patients. It may be worthwhile to try this treatment in severe cases of RSD with peripheral nerve damage such as seen in diabetic neuropathy.

TABLE 42a
RSD Types among 482 Consecutive Patients Suffering
from Chronic Pain followed over 5 Years[a]

RSD of disuse	82
Ephaptic RSD	19
	Total 101
Minor causalgia	11
Major causalgia	8

[a] To determine the incidence without thermography, the figure should be
approximately divided by four.

TABLE 42b
Outcome of Treatment in 101 Patients followed
5 Years or Longer

RSD of disuse	
Recovery (80–100% relief)	39
Partial improvement (over 50% relief)	18
Minimal relief	6
No relief	19
	Total 82
Ephaptic RSD	
Total recovery (including six morphine pump patients)	7
Partial improvement (one sympathectomy patient)[a]	8
No improvement (two sympathectomy patients)[a]	4
	Total 19

[a] Six more of these patients have undergone morphine pump treatment in the
past 2 years with total pain relief.

CONCLUSION

RSD is not an uncommon form of chronic pain. It has a variety of etiologies other than
trauma. It may originate in the periphery — face, neck, extremities, or trunk — or in the spinal
cord, brain stem, or cerebral hemispheres.

RSD has a variety of clinical manifestations from headache to muscle contraction, tremor,
or dystonia.

If any success is expected in treatment of RSD, the following multidisciplinary measures
should be applied:

1.   Early diagnosis before the sixth month after the original injury. This can be achieved by
an alert physician who realizes that one can rarely make an early diagnosis at the bedside
without tests.
Thermography is useful only in early diagnosis of RSD. It is not the diagnostic tool of
choice in identifying nerve roots damage. It is quite helpful in the diagnosis of atypical
RSD such as facial or cervicogenic RSD. Recognizing RSD originated from the cervical
spine region with the help of thermography spares the patient from unnecessary surgical
procedures for misdiagnosed conditions such as carpal tunnel syndrome, tardy ulnar
palsy, rotator cuff tear, thoracic outlet syndrome, and TMJ disease.
Bone scan is the second best tool in the diagnosis of RSD.

2. Early physiotherapy. As soon as the patient is diagnosed as suffering from RSD, extensive physical therapy (PT) at home and at the PT department is essential for success of treatment.

   Nerve block treatment should be combined with physiotherapy to ensure success.

   As early as possible, the patient should get rid of canes, walkers, crutches, braces, casts, wheelchairs, or any other assistive devices. The patient should return to work as soon as possible. Working is therapeutic for RSD patients.

3. Nerve block. Early application of nerve blocks in the hands of an experienced anesthesiologist substantially increases the success rate in treatment of RSD.

4. The above three criteria (early diagnosis, early physiotherapy, and early nerve blocks) should be complemented with discontinuation of narcotics, benzodiazepines, and barbiturates.

   The treatment of choice for chronic pain, especially in the form of RSD, is antidepressants, which are analgesic. Antidepressants that do not cause orthostatic hypotension or poor erection should be used. One example of the kind of antidepressant that helps such patients is Trazodone. In addition to being an analgesic for chronic pain, it increases REM sleep and, as a result, raises the pain threshold.

5. Sympatholytic medications as well as β- and calcium channel blockers are quite helpful in treatment of RSD. Propranolol should not be used because it aggravates depression as well as poor erection.

   Yohimbin, an α_2-blocker, timolol, a β-blocker, and the family of calcium channel blockers are quite helpful in the management of RSD.

   Judicious application of a strong α_1-blocker, phenoxybenzamine (Diabenzaline) is quite effective in the management of RSD.

6. By and large, invasive surgical procedures do not help RSD, and aggravate this form of chronic pain.

   Tractotomy, rhizotomy, cingulotomy, or any destructive procedure in CNS inevitably fail and usually aggravate RSD.

   Spinal cord stimulators are no different than transcutaneous nerve stimulators (TNS), and after a few months the brain ignores the repetitive digital stimulation by such devices. Subsequently the patient is left with a foreign body in the spinal canal that becomes a new source of chronic pain.

7. Sympathectomy should be reserved only for patients who have a very short life expectancy (less than 5 years). In patients who are expected to live longer than 5 years, sympathectomy takes away the natural temperature regulation system and leaves the patient vulnerable to exaggeration of chronic pain of RSD by any minor climatic change.

8. None of the above treatments will succeed unless the patient is taken off alcohol, narcotics, benzodiazepines, and foods rich in tyrosine, nitrites, and phenethylamine (chocolate).

   Only one physician should be in charge of the medications, with the main goal being detoxification from BZs and narcotics.

9. The teamwork of neurologists, physiatrists, and anesthesiologists is necessary for successful treatment.

Objective neuropsychometric tests are quite helpful in the management of these patients. However, these can be done by a psychologist. If the disease is diagnosed and treated early, usually there is no need for a psychiatrist to be involved.

Above all, health care providers who are expected to treat these patients should be excused from the care of these patients and involvement in treatment if they have a biased view of chronic pain patients. If physicians consider chronic pain patients as "malingerers", "primary or secondary gain individuals", or "psychotics", their body language shows their hostility toward the patient, and treatment is guaranteed to fail.

RECENT ADVANCES AND FUTURE TRENDS

EARLY DIAGNOSIS

Worldwide, researchers are emphasizing the importance of early diagnosis and early treatment in the management of RSD.[493-500] Application of thermography is the key to early diagnosis. Stage 1 and early stage 2 RSD is usually easy to treat with a high rate of success.

Early diagnosis seems to play a more important role than the mode of treatment in the outcome of the management of RSD.

DIAGNOSTIC METHODS

Thermography seems to be the most sensitive test for early diagnosis of RSD.[501-503] Bennett and Ochoa[503] demonstrated that this method can be used in experimental animal models in the study and diagnosis of RSD.

Another test that seems to be quite promising in diagnosis and management of RSD is Doppler flow study of the extremity.[505] This method measures changes in the skin capillary blood flow (SBF). The temperature before, during, and 1 hour after unilateral lumbar paravertebral sympathetic block was studied simultaneously with laser Doppler flowmetry and thermometry in patients with RSD. This method was useful in the detection of immediate onset of sympathetic block in patients who were undergoing sympathetic block under anesthesia and who could not verbally identify relief with the block due to anesthesia or conscious sedation.[505]

Bej and Schwartzman[506] evaluated the response of cutaneous blood flow to autonomic stimuli in eight patients in different stages of RSD. They compared these results with eight healthy controlled subjects. They measured the blood flow in the affected and contralateral extremities by laser Doppler fluxmetry. They applied five autonomic stimuli to the contralateral extremity during blood flow measurement in the ipsilateral diseased extremity.

They found that the limb afflicted by RSD had lost the normal reflex reduction of blood flow in the extremity with the Valsalva maneuver and with cold response test. The normal contralateral limb did show the proper normal response as mentioned above.

They did not notice any differences in the baseline blood flow between patients and controls, nor did they find any difference of temperature of the extremities between the patients and controls. This may be explained by the fact that in both normal and RSD individuals the skin temperature and deep visceral temperature fluctuate depending on how active the sympathetic nervous system is. The more active the sympathetic system, the colder the surface temperature and warmer the deeper visceral temperature, and vice versa. So the total balance of temperature and blood flow usually stays stable.

The diseased RSD extremity also lacked the rhythmic cycling of cutaneous blood flow that typifies the normal extremity. They emphasized the importance of the efferent sympathetic system in causation of RSD.[506]

Similarly, McMahon[507] pointed to the efferent sympathetic system perpetuating the sympathetically maintained pain (SMP).[508] He emphasized that the normal tissue activity in postganglionic sympathetic efferents does not produce pain, nor is it capable of activating nociceptive sensory neurons. It can, however, induce modest firing in some mechanoreceptors. SMP results from a vicious circle of events, which includes changes in peripheral and central somatosensory processes, most importantly due to a positive feedback element in the form of sympathetic efferent neurons activating sensory neurons peripherally, completing the vicious circle of sympathetic hyperactivity and perpetuation of sympathetic maintained pain.[507]

However, the peripheral pathology completing the vicious circle cannot be ignored. The disruption of efferent sympathetic modulation results in supersensivity of sensory end organs to norepinephrine.[509] This end organ supersensitivity, which may explain the reason for failure of sympathectomy in relieving sympathetic pain, is due to α_1-adrenergic receptors' supersensitivity.[509,510] Norepinephrine and dihydroxyphenylethylene glycol (DHPG) activate the α_1

sensory receptors, resulting in peripheral vascular constriction.[509,510] On the other hand, sympathetic nerve block deactivates this phenomenon.

This explains why clonidine, an α_2-blocker, and propranolol, a β-blocker, are not effective in relief of sympathetically mediated pain (SMP);[510] whereas, α_1-blockers are quite effective in the relief of SMP and vasoconstriction.

OTHER ADVANCES IN DIAGNOSTIC METHODS
Bone Scan

As is well known, technetium-99 scintigraphy can show confusing results in different stages of RSD. In Stage I, as expected, the bone scan shows an increased blood flow in the involved joint, whereas in Stages II and III it may show a decreased flow in the involved joint.[511] This explains the confusing results on bone scan. Not infrequently, the attention is concentrated on the area of increased uptake of the technetium, whereas in the contralateral extremity it is the source of the pathology and is showing a relative decreased flow due to the later stages of RSD.

MRI

The diagnostic use of magnetic resonance imaging (MRI) in RSD usually is not informative.[512] Even though MRI is reported to be slightly more sensitive than bone scan,[30] advocates of MRI for this disease admit to its limitation and to the higher cost involved in performing MRI for the diagnosis of RSD.[513]

It is obvious that by the time anatomical tests such as X-rays, CT scan, or MRI show areas of density changes in the bone, the disease is quite advanced, and the diagnosis can be more accurately made by other methods such as bone scan[511] or thermography.[514–516]

MRI is useful mainly to rule out other causes of pain, but its use as a diagnostic tool in RSD is limited and especially costly.[513]

Doppler flow study[505, 506] can be quite helpful in the diagnosis of RSD.

FURTHER ADVANCES IN ETIOLOGY OF RSD

Some unlikely causes are added to the long list of etiology of RSD. In patients who have renal transplant and require cyclosporin-A, the use of large doses or cyclosporin-A causes RSD around the joints. This is dose related, and reduction of the dose of cyclosporin-A corrects this condition.[517]

Similarly, the use of ergot medications such as given for patients suffering from headaches can initiate RSD.[518] This is important because of the fact that a lot of craniofacial injuries can initiate RSD, and the use of ergot medications is quite common in such patients. As a result, this iatrogenic factor aggravates the tendency for RSD and deterioration of the patient's headaches.

This RSD may be due to persistence of irritation of lumbar nerve roots after surgery. An extruded disc fragment — laterally positioned and missed at the time of surgery — can cause and perpetuate RSD in the distribution of the irritated nerve root.[519]

Nerve root compression similarly can cause RSD in the distribution of lumbar nerve roots.[520] These examples are added to the not uncommon complication of RSD due to contusion of nerve roots that have already been discussed in previous chapters.

Another postoperative form of RSD is RSD after podiatric surgery[521] or plastic surgery. This is not at all uncommon and can be in two forms:

1.   In the first form, the patient who has RSD due to an old nerve damage, podiatric surgery in this area causes new scar formation and severe ephaptic RSD.
     One such example seen in our practice is a patient who suffered from multiple sclerosis, which was in remission for a few decades. One residual of the disease was a sustained Babinski. The podiatrist tried to operate on the first toe to get rid of the deformity, which

he diagnosed as "hammer toe". This not only caused further deformity of the extended big toe, but caused RSD.

2. Another area of high risk regarding development of postoperative RSD is hand plastic surgery. Dupuytran syndrome and its surgical correction can lead to RSD.[522] RSD may develop after carpal tunnel syndrome surgery.[523,524] Some of the factors in the development of RSD may be a tendency for variations in sympathetic nervous system fibers in the trunk of median nerve,[523] as well as not exposing and complete decompression of the median nerve at the time of surgery.[523,524]

    Another factor that we have noticed quite commonly is confusing RSD involving the wrist and hand for carpal tunnel syndrome and performing surgery in the area already affected by RSD, with disastrous results.

CANCER AND RSD

Malignancy is a well-known etiology of RSD, as mentioned in the Chapter 9 on Etiology. A recent study[525] confirms this phenomenon.

MANIFESTATIONS OF DIFFERENT STAGES OF RSD

In Stage I, an indulated skin edema may be the sole manifestation of development of RSD.[526]

In Stage III, efferent hyperactivity and motor deformity in the form of movement disorder, flexion deformity, tremor, and other manifestations that have already been discussed in detail can be the main disabling factors in RSD.[528]

HEADACHE AND RSD

A rare form of vascular headache, episodic paroxysmal hemicrania (EPH), which causes unilateral headache, ipsilateral conjunctivitis, and frequently Horner's syndrome and rhinorrhea, has been reported to respond quite favorably to calcium channel blockers.[543]

Realizing that EPH is very difficult to treat, it is encouraging that Coria and colleagues[543] have had such good results with calcium channel blockers (see Table 20 and Figure 18a).

DERMATOLOGIC MANIFESTATIONS OF RSD

Usually in the late stages of RSD, skin eruptions and other dermatologic manifestations are complicated by the clinical picture of RSD.

Reticulate hyperpigmentation, xerosis, neurodermatitis, plaque formation, and skin eruptions in the distal portion of the extremity are some common dermatologic manifestations of late RSD.[527] On the other hand, cutaneous atrophy and elephantiasis are some rare dermatologic forms of RSD.

Whenever there is a persistence of neurodermatitis in the distribution of a dermatome or thermatome that does not clear up with standard treatments and has a tendency for recurrence, one should suspect RSD as the etiology.

PREGNANCY AND RSD

RSD seems to be affecting pregnant women more commonly than other patients.[528,529] This is seen in the form of focal and rapid osteoporosis in different bones, especially the hips.[528,529] The hormonal changes during pregnancy have been blamed for this complications.[529] However, another factor may be a tendency for inactivity toward the end of pregnancy.

Usually the RSD complicating pregnancy corrects itself after delivery and child birth.

SHOULDER PAIN AND RSD

Involvement of shoulder pathology in RSD and vice versa is quite common. The involvement of the shoulder is a reflection of multiple causes[545] as follows:

1. Local pathology around the shoulder joint can instigate the development of RSD.
2. Referred pain, such as in the case of heart attack, can cause limitation of motion of the shoulder and the development of RSD.
3. Shoulder pain may be a reflection of direct involvement of the nerves being irritated in the cervical spine, such as in the case of cervical sprain, cervical spondylosis, or cervical disc herniation.
4. RSD involving the upper extremity quite commonly causes limitation of motion of the shoulder and involvement of the shoulder in RSD.[530]

Regardless of the cause, local chemical blocks around the shoulder joints are quite successful in the management of RSD involving the shoulder joint.

Injection of suprascapular nerve[531] as well as repeated injections of trigger points around the shoulder are quite helpful and result in excellent relief of shoulder immobility and shoulder pain.

The patient may require repeated injections or at times even continuous stellate block injection.[539] This continuous stellate block injection has been reported to have a success rate of up to 75% even in the advanced stages of RSD.[532]

As it has been repeatedly emphasized, injections around the shoulder joints have to be followed by aggressive physiotherapy; injections alone cannot be relied on to cure RSD with shoulder involvement.

REGIONAL SYMPATHETIC BLOCK

Sympathetic block seems to be the most effective form of treatment for RSD. Again, early diagnosis and early administration of the block are the key to success of the treatment.[493–497]

If the diagnosis is made within the first 3 months of onset of RSD and if the block is applied in the first 3 months, the rate of success will be much higher.

In this regard, awareness of RSD as the etiology of chonic pain and application of sensitive tests such as thermography and bone scan[544] and Doppler study[505] applied within the first 2 to 3 months are essential. Early diagnosis followed by early block are imperative for success of the treatment.[497,533]

At times the blocks are quite successful if they are aimed at the area of the nerve that originates the pathology. Examples are suprascapular nerve block,[531] and injection in the area of brachial plexus when the pathology is distal to the brachial plexus.[534] Epidural blocks are also quite helpful.[493,494]

REGITINE TEST

Intravenous phentolamine (regitine) is a good test to detect the potential efficacy of guanethidine block.[535] This test in patients in whom the pain was transiently relieved by i.v. regitine showed subsequent sympathalytic treatment with i.v. regional guanethaline had more favorable and successful results. This test should be considered before the patient undergoes the tedious and painful i.v. guanethaline block.[535]

OTHER FORMS OF TREATMENT

Oral intake of antiinflammatory medications may be helpful in the treatment of RSD, but it is not enough.[536] One antiinflammatory medication, ketrolac (Tolmetin or Toredal®), can help relieve the symptoms of RSD.[537]

As mentioned earlier, capsaicin is quite helpful in the relief of painful RSD, especially in disease such as diabetic neuropathy and postherpetic neuropathy.[538]

Calcitonin has been tried in the treatment of focal osteoporosis due to RSD.[539,540] However, this treatment is not effective mainly because it simply tries to correct the effect rather than the cause of the disease.

The use of RU486 is not limited to birth control. It blocks cortisol receptors and raises the levels of ACTH and endorphins secreted by pituitary.[244] This phenomenon may be beneficial in treatment of depression, as well as in narcotic detoxification.

OPIOID WITHDRAWAL

Opioid withdrawal in the acute stage results in hyperactivity of the sympathetic system and manifestation of a clinical picture identical to RSD.[541]

It becomes obvious that as long as the patient is on oral i.m. narcotics, every 3 to 4 hours the body is challenged with opioid withdrawal and resultant aggravation of RSD.

Therefore, the first goal should be discontinuation of oral i.m. opioids in the management of RSD.

It is suggested by Hannington-Kiff that natural opioid peptide modulation in regional sympathetic ganglia normally rises to prevent excessive autonomic activity in an injured limb.[541] The regional nature of natural opioid modulation (dynorphin) on regional sympathetic ganglia is quite preventive, but it is counteracted by the use of exorphins (oral i.m. narcotics). Such use prevents the regional formation of dynorphins, and as a result causes hypersensitivity of the limb for development of RSD.

SYMPATHECTOMY

The interest in sympathectomy has not been phased out among vascular surgeons.

Olcott et al.[542] report results of sympathectomy among 35 patients performed in a period of 3.5 years on the basis of at least one positive diagnostic sympathetic block. The patients were followed for only 1 to 4 months. They report excellent results in 74%, good results in 17%, and poor results in 9% of these patients. Three patients required a repeat cervical sympathectomy after the initial surgery failed to relieve the pain. One patient required a contralateral lumbar sympathectomy. They believe that if the patient does not respond to sympathectomy, further sympathectomy by an alternate approach should be tried for further removal of the residual sympathetic tissue.

This report again repeats the optimistic results of sympathectomy in short-term followups (1–4 months). It remains to be seen how many of these excellent and good results of sympathectomy will be retained after 5 to 10 years.

Procedures such as extensive sympathectomy and especially bilateral lumbar sympathectomy[542] are quite disabling for the patient because of the severe orthostatic hypotension and other complications of extensive sympathectomy.

The general trend is avoidance of sympathectomy except for patients who have a short life (5 years or less) expectancy — such as in the cases of cancer and advanced diabetes.

Morphine pump is the successful procedure of last resort if all fails.

FUTURE TRENDS

The future trend seems to be in terms of early diagnosis, early nerve block, early aggressive treatment, early physiotherapy, and, more importantly, prevention of RSD by avoiding unnecessary surgery and unnecessary invasive procedures, especially in the parts of body such as the hand, foot, and knee where there is more of a tendency for the development of RSD.

The importance of discontinuation of narcotics and benzodiazepines in the management of RSD cannot be overemphasized.

Awareness of the unusual and peculiar manifestations such as movement disorders, emotional hyperpathic pain, and dermatologic complications by frontline physicians (ER doctors, orthopedists, and plastic surgeons) and postgraduate training of such physicians in the subject of complex chronic pain (CCP) are essential in the prevention and management of RSD pain; most importantly, this teaches them not to use narcotics on such patients and helps them develop empathy for and understanding of the complex chronic pain (CCP) of sympathetic mediated pain (SMP) also called RSD.

References

1. Abram, S. E., Asiddao, C. B., and Reynolds, A. C. Increased skin temperature during transcutaneous electrical stimulation. *Anesth. Analg.* 59:22–25, 1980.
2. Abram, S. E. and Lightfoot, R. W. Treatment of longstanding causalgia with prazosin. *Reg. Anaesth.* 6:79–81, 1981.
3. Adams, R. D. and Victor, M. *Principles of Neurology*, 3rd ed., New York: McGraw-Hill, 1985.
4. Adler, I. Muscular rheumatism. *Med. Rec.* 57:529–535, 1900.
5. Aghajanian, G. K. and Wang, R. Y. Physiology and pharmacology of central serotonergic neurons. In Lipton, M. A., DiMascio, A., and Killiam, K. F., eds. *Psychopharmacology: A Generation of Progress*. New York: Raven Press, 1978.
6. Albe-Fessard, D. and Lombard, M. D. Use of an animal model to evaluate the origin of and protection against deafferentation pain. Bonica, J. J., ed. In *Proceedings of the Third World Congress on Pain*. New York: Raven Press, 1983. *Adv. Pain Res.Ther.* 691–700, 1983.
7. Albert, M. I. Carbamazepine for painful post-traumatic paresthesiae. *N. Engl. J. Med.* 290:693, 1974.
8. Albritten, F. F. and Maltby, G. L. Causalgia secondary to injury of the major peripheral nerves: Treatment by sympathectomy. *Surgery* 19:407–414, 1946.
9. An, H. S., Hawthorne, K. B., et al. Reflex sympathetic dystrophy and cigarette smoking. *J. Hand Surg.* (3), May, 1988.
10. Andersson, K. E. and Vinge, E. Beta-adrenoceptor blockers and calcium antagonists in the prophylaxis and treatment of migraine. *Drugs* 39(3):355–373, 1990.
11. Anthony, M. The biochemistry of migraine. Rose, F. C., ed. In *Handbook of Clinical Neurology*, Vol 48. Amsterdam: Elsevier Science, 1986.
12. Arner, S., Meyerson, B., and Persson, H. Intravenous regional sympathetic blockade with guanethidine. *Opuscula Med.* 25(4):128–132, 1980. (In Swedish.)
13. Ashwal, S. Reflex sympathetic dystrophy syndrome in children, *Pediatr. Neurol.* 4(1):38, 1988.
14. Bajorek, J. G., Lee, R. J., and Lomax, K. Neuropeptides: Anticonvulsant and convulsant mechanisms in epileptic model systems and in humans. *Adv. Neurol.* 44:489–500, 1986.
15. Baker, A. G. and Wingarner, F. G. Causalgia, A review of twenty-eight treated cases. *Am. J. Surg.* 117:690–694, 1969.
16. Barasi, S. and Lynn, B. Effects of sympathetic stimulation on mechanoreceptor and nociceptor afferent units with small myelinated (A-delta) and unmyelinated (C) axons innervating the rabbit pinna. *J. Physiol. (London)* 341:51P, 1983.
17. Barnes, R. The role of sympathectomy in the treatment of causalgia. *J. Bone Joint Surg. (Br.)* 35B:172–180, 1953.
18a. Barré, M. J. Sur un syndrome sympathique cervical posterieur et sa cause frequent, l'artrite cervical. *Rev. Neurol. Paris* 1:1246–1248, 1926.
18b. Lieou, Y. C. Syndrome sympathique cervical posterieur et arthrite cervical chronique, etude clinique et radiologique, Strasbourgh, 1928 (Thesis).
19. Barolat, G., Schwartzman, R., et al. Epidural spinal cord stimulation in the management of reflex sympathetic dystrophy. *Stereotact. Funct. Neurosurg.* 53:29–39, 1989.
20. Bayless, W. M. On the origin from the spinal cord of the vasodilator fibres of the hind limb and on the nature of these fibres. *J. Physiol.* 26:173–209, 1901.
21. Beck, L. Histamine as the potential mediator for active reflex dilation. *Fed. Proc.* 24:1298–1310, 1965.
22. Bej, M. D. and Schwartzman, R. J. Abnormalities of cutaneous blood flow regulation in patients with reflex sympathetic dystrophy as measured by laser Doppler fluxmetry. *Arch. Neurol.* 48:912–915, 1991.
23. Bell, C. and Auton, J. Vasadilator neurons supplying skin and skeletal muscles of limbs. *J. Auton. Nerv. Syst.* 7:257–262, 1938.
24. Benzon, H. T., Chomka, C. M., and Brunner, E. A. Treatment of reflex sympathetic dystrophy with regional intravenous reserpine. *Anesth. Analg.* 59:500–502, 1980.
25. Berguer, R. and Smith, R. Transaxillary sympathectomy (T2 to T4) for relief of vasospastic/sympathetic pain of upper extremities. *Surgery* 89:764–769, 1981.
26. Bernad, P. G. and Perio, V. P. Horner syndrome with causalgia. *Neurology* 30:534–535, 1980.

27. Bernstein, B. H., Singsen, B. H., Kent, J. T., et al. Reflex neurovascular dystrophy in childhood. *J. Pediatr.* 93:211–215, 1978.
28. Bier, A. Uber einen neuen Weg Lokalanesthesie an den Gliedmassen zu Erzeugen. Verhandlungen der Deutschen Gesellschaft fur Chirurgie 37 (2):204, 1908.
29. Bjorklund, A. and Hokfelt, T. *Handbook of Chemical Neuroanatomy.* Amsterdam: Elsevier, 1983, pp. 176–177.
30. Bloom, F. E., Battenberg, E., Rosier, J., Ling, N., and Guillemin, R. Neurons containing B-endorphin in rat brain exist separately from those containing enkephalin: Immunocytochemical studies. *Proc. Natl. Acad. Sci. U.S.A.* 75:1591–1595, 1978.
31. Bloom, F. E., Battenberg, E. L. F., Shibasaki, T., Benoit, R., Ling, N., and Guillemin, R. Localization of v-melanocyte stimulating hormone (M. S. H.) immunoreactivity in rat brain and pituitary. *Regul. Pept.* 1:205–222, 1980.
32. Blumberg, H. and Janig, W. Activation of fibers via experimentally-produced stump neuromas in skin nerves: Ephaptic transmissions or retrograde sprouting? *Exp. Neurol.* 76:468–482, 1982.
33. Blumberg, H. and Janig, W. Discharge patterns of afferent fibers from a neuroma. *Pain* 20(4):335–353, 1984.
34. Botney, M. and Fields, H. L. Amitriptyline potentiates morphine analgesia by a direct action on the central nervous system. *Ann. Neurol.* 13:160–164, 1983.
35. Bondarchuck, A. V. (Surgical treatment of causalgia of the upper limbs.) Vaprosy nevrokhirurgii. *Moscow* 8(3):37, 1944.
36. Bonica, J. J. Causalgia and other sympathetic dystrophies. In *Advances in Pain Research and Therapy.* New York: Raven Press, 1979, pp. 141–146, 177.
37. Bonica, J. J. Causalgia and other reflex sympathetic dystrophies. *Postgrad. Med.* 53:143–148, 1973.
38. Bonica, J. J. *The Management of Pain,* Vol. 1, 2nd ed., Philadelphia: Lea & Febiger, 1990, p. 236.
39. Bonica, J. J. *The Management of Pain.* Philadelphia: Lea & Febiger, 1990, p. 228.
40. Bonica, J. J. *The Management of Pain.* Philadelphia: Lea & Febiger, 1953.
41. Bonica, J. J. *Sympathetic Nerve Blocks for Pain Diagnosis and Therapy,* Vol. 1. New York: Breon Laboratories, 1980, pp. 27–38.
42. Bonner, R. F., Clem, T. R., Bowen, P. D., and Bowman, R. L. Laser Doppler continuous real-time monitor of pulsatile and mean blood flow in tisue microcirculation Chen, S.-H., Chu, B., and Norral, R., eds. In *Scattering Techniques Applied to Supramolecular and Nonequilirium Systems.* New York: Plenum Press, 1981, pp. 685–701.
43. Bonner, R. F., Nossal, R., Havlin, S., and Weiss, G. H. Model for photon migration in turbid biological media. *J. Opt. Soc. Am.* Vol. A 4:423–432, 1987.
44. Bossi, L., Conoscente, F., et al. Algodystrophy: Treatment. *Funct. Neurol.* 4(2):157, 1989.
45. Bowman, W. C. Effects of adrenergic activators and inhibitors on the skeletal muscles. Szekeres L., ed. In *Handbook of Experimental Pharmacology,* Vol. 54(pt. 2) New York: Springer-Verlag, 1981, pp. 47–128.
46. Brand, P. W. and Curtis, R. M. The imbalanced hand and the stiff hand, II. Conservative management and surgical treatment of the stiff hand. Instructional course given at the annual meeting of The American Academy of Orthopaedic Surgeons, New Orleans, Louisiana, February 1, 1976.
47. Brattberg, G., Thorslund, M., and Wikman, A. The validity of a pain questionnaire for postal surveys. *Clin. J. Pain* 6:199–205, 1990.
48. Breivik, H. Intravenous sympathetic blockade with guanethidine. *Tidsskr Nor Laegeforen* 99:935–939, 1979. (In Norwegian.)
49. Brock, T. R. Reflex sympathetic dystrophy linked to venipuncture: A case report. *J. Oral Maxillofac Surg.* 47:1333–1335, 1989.
50. Brown, R., Bassett, L. W., Wexler, C. E., et al. Thermography as a screening modality for nerve fiber irritation in patients with low back pain: A pilot study. Modern Medicine, Special Supplement; Academy of Neuro-Muscular Thermography. *Clin. Proc.* September: pp. 86–88, 1987.
51. Buker, R. H., Cox, W. A., Scully, T. J., et al. Causalgia and transthoracic sympathectomy. *Am. J. Surg.* 724–727, 1972.
52. Burchiel, K. J. and Russell, L. C. Spontaneous activity of ventral root axons following peripheral nerve injury. *J. Neurosurg.* 62:408–413, 1985.
53. Buzzi, M. G. and Moskowitz, M. A. The antimigraine drug, sumatriptan (GR43175), selectively blocks neurogenic plasma extravasation from blood vessels in dura mater. *Br. J. Pharmacol.* 99:202–206, 1990.
54. Campbell, J. M. and Jaces, C. Lesions in the region of the dorsal root entry zone (DREZ) relieve pain from avulsion of the brachial plexus (Abstract). American Pain Society, 5th General Meeting, Dallas, 1985.
55. Carter, H. W. On causalgia and applied painful conditions due to lesions of the peripheral nerves. *J. Neurol. Psychopathol.* 3:l, 1922.
56. Casale, R. and LaRovere, M. T. Increased sympathetic tone in the left arm of patients affected by symptomatic myocardial ischemia. *Funct. Neurol.* 4(2):161, 1989.
57. Casten, D. F. and Betcher, A. M. Reflex sympathetic dystrophy, *Surg. Gynecol. Obstet.* 100:97–100, 1955.

58. Celander, O. and Folkow, B. A comparison of the sympathetic vasomotor fibre control of the vessels within the skin and the muscles. *Acta Physiol. Scand.* 29:241–250, 1953.

59. Chafetz, N., Wexler, C. E., and Kaiser, J. A. Neuromuscular thermography of the lumbar spine with CT correlation. *Spine* 13:(8) pp. 922–925, 1988.

60. Chaturvedi, S. K. Phenytoin in reflex sympathetic dystrophy, *Pain* 36:379–380, 1989.

61. Chernetski, K. E. Sympathetic enhancement of peripheral sensory input in the frog. *J. Neurophysiol.* 27:493–515, 1964.

62. Chostine, S. Y., Comair, Y. G., Turner, D. M., et al. Phenoxybenzamine in the treament of causalgia: Report of 40 cases. *J. Neurosurg.* 60:1263–1268, 1984.

63. Cicuttini, F. and Littlejohn, G. E. Female adolescent rheumatological presentations: The importance of chronic pain syndromes, *Aust. Paediatr. J.* 25:21–24, 1989.

64. Cline, M. A., Ochoa, J., and Torebjork, E. Chronic Hyperalgesia and Skin Warming Caused by Sensitized C Nociceptors, *Brain* 112:621–647, 1989.

65. Cohen, S. *The Chemical Brain. The Neurochemistry of Addictive Disorders.* Compcare Institute, Irvine, CA, 1988.

66. Conant, J., Engler, R., et al. Central nervous system side effects of beta-adrenergic blocking agents with high and low lipid solubility. *J. Cardiovasc. Pharmacol.* 13:656–661, 1989.

67. Cooke, E. D. and Ward, C. Vicious circles in reflex sympathetic dystrophy — a hypothesis: Discussion paper. *J. R. Soc. Med.* 83:96, 1990.

68. Cooper, D. E., DeLee, J. C., et al. Reflex sympathetic dystrophy of the knee. *J. Bone Joint Surg.* 71-A(3), 1989.

69. Coppack, S. W. and Watkins, P. J. The natural history of diabetic femoral neuropathy. *Q. J. Med.* 79:307–313, 1991.

70. Young et al. Corticotropin releasing hormone stimulation. *Mayo Clinic Proc.* 65:945–946, 1990.

71. Cremer, S. A., Maynard, F., and Davidoff, G. The reflex sympathetic dystrophy syndrome associated with traumatic myelopathy: Report of 5 cases. *Pain* 37:187–192, 1989.

72. Dale, W. A. and Lewis, M. R. Management of ischemia of the hand and fingers. *Surgery* 67:62, 1970.

73. Davidoff, G., Morey, K., Amann, M., et al. Pain measurement in reflex sympathetic dystrophy syndrome. *Pain* 32:27–34, 1988.

74. Davies, K. H. Guanethidine sympathetic blockade: Its value in reimplantation surgery. *Br. Med. J.* 876, 1976.

75. Davis, S. W., et al. Shoulder-hand syndrome in a hemiplegic population: 5-year retrospective study. *Arch. Phys. Med. Rehabil.* 58:3553, 1977.

76. Daw, N. W., Rader, R. K., Robertson, T. W., et al. Effects of 6-hydroxydopamine on visual deprivation in the kitten striate cortex. *J. Neurosci.* 3:907–941, 1983.

77. Demangeat, J., Constantinesco, A., et al. Three-Phase bone scanning in reflex sympathetic dystrophy of the hand. *J. Nucl. Med.* 29:26–32, 1988.

78. Dent, C. E. and Friedman, M. Idiopathic juvenile osteoporosis. *Q. J. Med.* 34:177, 1965.

79. DeTakats, G. Reflex dystrophy of the extremities, *Arch. Surg.* 34:939–956, 1937.

80. Devor, M. The pathophysiology and anatomy of damaged nerve. Wall, P. D., Melzack, R., eds. In *Textbook of Pain.* New York: Churchill Livingston, 1984, pp. 49–64.

81. Devor, M. Nerve pathophysiology and mechanisms of pain in causalgia. *J. Auton. Nerv. Sys.* 7:371–384, 1983.

82. Devor, M. and Janig, L. W. Activation of myelinated afferent ending in a neuroma by stimulation of the sympathetic supply in the rat. Neurosci. Lett. 24:43–47, 1981.

83. Devor, M. and Wall, P. D. Effect of peripheral nerve injury on receptive field of cells in the cat spinal cord. *J. Comp. Neurol.* 199:277–291, 1981.

84. Doupe, J., Cullen, C. H., and Chance, G. W. Post-traumatic pain and the causalgic syndrome. *J. Neurol. Neurosurg. Psychiat.* 7:33–48, 1944.

85. Doury, P. Algodystrophy, reflex sympathetic dystrophy syndrome. *Clin. Rheumatol.* 7(2):173–180, 1988.

86. Drucker, W. R., Hubay, C. A., Holden, W. D., et al. Pathogenesis of post-traumatic sympathetic dystrophy. *Am. J. Surg.* 97:454–465, 1959.

87. Duensing, F., Becker, P., and Rittmeyer, K. Thermographic findings in lumbar disc protrusions. *Arch. Psychiatr. Nervenkr.* 217:53–70, 1973.

88. Duncan, K. H., Lewis, R. C., et al. Treatment of upper extremity reflex sympathetic dystrophy with joint stiffness using sympatholytic bier blocks and manipulation. *Orthopedics* II(6):883, 1988.

89. Echlin, F., Owens, F. M., et al. Observations on "major" and "minor" causalgia. *Arch. Neurol. Psychiat.* 62:183, 1949.

90. Elfvin, L. G., and Dalsgaard, C. J. Retrograde axonal transport of horseradish peroxidase in afferent fibers of the inferior mesenteric ganglion of the guinea-pig. Identification of the cells of origin in dorsal root ganglia. *Brain Res.* 126:149–153, 1977.

91. Emson, P. C. *Chemical Neuroanatomy.* New York: Raven Press, 1983, p. 167.

92. Emson, P. C. *Chemical Neuroanatomy.* New York: Raven Press, 1983, pp. 177–184.

93. Ertekin, C., et al. Chiappa, K. H., ed. In *Evoked Potentials in Clinical Medicine.* New York: Raven Press, 1983, p. 285.

94. Escobar, P. L. Reflex sympathetic dystrophy, *Orthop. Rev.* 15:646–651, 1986.

95. Evans, J. A. Reflex sympathetic dystrophy: Report on 57 cases. *Ann. Intern. Med.* 26:417–426, 1947.

96. Fagrell, B., Froneck, A., and Intaglietta, M. A microscope television system for dynamic studies of blood flow velocity in human skin capillaries. *Am. J. Physiol.* 233:H318 21, 1977.

97. Fischer, A. Diagnosis and management of chronic pain in physical medicine and rehabilitation. Ruskin, A. P. ed. In *Current Therapy in Psychiatry.* Philadelphia: W. B. Saunders, 1984, pp. 123–145.

98. Fischer, A. The present status of neuromuscular thermography. Academy of Neuro-Muscular Thermography, first annual meeting, May 1985; postgraduate Medicine 1986; special edition pp. 26–33.

99. Fischer, A., Rim, A., and Chang, C. Correlation between thermographic findings and somatosensory cortical evoked potentials in lumbosacral radiculopathies. *Thermology* 2:29–33, 1986.

100. Foley, D., Schatz, L., et al. Topical nitroglycerin facilitats intravenous regional techniques in patients with reflex sympathetic dystrophy. *Anesthesiology* 69:1029, 1988.

101. Folkow, B. Nervous control of blood vessels. *Acta Physiol. Scand.* 35:629–663, 1955.

102. Foster, O., Askaria, A., Lanham, J., et al. Algoneurodystrophy following herpes zoster. *Postgrad. Med. J.* 65:478–480, 1989.

103. Fox, R. H. and Edholm, O. G. Nervous control of the cutaneous circulation. *Br. Med. Bull.* 19:110–114, 1963.

104. Fraser, R. and Pare, J. Perception in chest roentgenology. In *Diagnosis of Diseases of the Chest*, 2nd ed. Philadelphia: W. B. Saunders, 1977.

105. Freeman, N. E. The treatment of causalgia arising from gunshot wounds of the peripheral nerves. *Surgery* 22:68, 1947.

106. Gandhavadi, B., Rosen, J. S., and Addison, R. C. Autonomic pain — features and methods of assessment. *Postgrad. Med.* 71:85–90, 1982.

107. Gaucher, A., et al. The diagnostic value of 99mTc-disphophonate bone imaging in transient osteoporosis of the hip. *J. Rheumatol.* 6:774, 1979.

108. Gavras, I., et al. A comparative study of the effects of oxprenolol versus propranolol in essential hypertension. *J. Clin. Pharmacol.* 19:8–14, 1979.

109. Gellman, H., Eckert, R. R., et al. Reflex sympathetic dystrophy in cervical spinal cord injury patients. *Clin. Orthopaed. Relat. Res.* (233), 1988.

110. Genant, H. K., et al. The reflex sympathetic dystrophy syndrome: A comprehensive analysis using fine-detail radiography, photon absorptiometry and bone and joint scintigraphy. *Radiology* 117:21, 1975.

111. Genant, H. K., et al. The reflex sympathetic dystrophy syndrome. *Radiology* 117:21, 1975.

112. Gillstrom, P. Thermography in low back pain and sciatica. *Arch. Orthop. Trauma Surg.* 104:31–36, 1985.

113. Gold, B., Brickner, D., et al. Reflex sympathetic dystrophy syndrome following minor trauma. *Israel J. Med. Sci.* 25, 1989.

114. Gold. P. W., Goodwin, F. K., et al. Clinical and biochemical manifestations of depression. *N. Eng. J. Med.* 319:7:413–420, 1988.

115. Golden, R. N., Hoffman, J., Falk, D., Provenzale, D., and Curtis, T. E. Psychoses associated with propranolol withdrawal. *Biol. Psychiat.* 25:351–354, 1989.

116. Good, M. Five hundred cases of myalgia in the British army. *Ann. Rheum. Dis.* 3:118–138, 1942.

117. Graham, C., Bond, S. S., Gerkovich, M. M., and Cook, M. R. Use of the McGill Pain Questionnaire in the assessment of cancer pain; replicability and consistency. *Pain* 8:377–387, 1980.

118. Granit, R., Leksell, L., and Skoglund, C. R. Fiber interaction in injured or compressed region of nerve. *Brain* 67:125–140, 1944.

119. Grefrath, S. P., Smith, P. B., and Appel, S. A. Characterization of the B2-adrenergic receptor and adenylate cyclase in skeletal muscle plasma membranes. *Arch. Biochem. Biophys.* 188:328–337, 1978.

120. Griffin, S. J. and Friedman, J. J. Depressive symptoms in propranolol users. *J. Clin. Psychiat.* 47:453–457, 1986.

121. Gross, D. Pain and autonomic nervous system. *Adv. Neurol.* 4:93–103, 1974.

122. Grunert, B. K., Devine, C. A., et al. Thermal self-regulation for pain control in reflex sympathetic dystrophy syndrome. *J. Hand Surg.* 15A:615–618, 1990.

123. Gutstein, M. Diagnosis and treatment of muscular rheumatism. *Br. J. Phys. Med.* 1:302–321, 1938.

124. Hagbarth, K. E. and Vallbo, A. B. Afferent response to mechanical stimulation of muscle receptors in man. *ACTA Soc. Med. Upsal* 72:102–114, 1967.

125. Hallin, R. G. and Wiesenfield-Hallin, A. Does sympathetic activity modify afferent inflow at the receptor level in man? *J. Auton. Nerv. Syst.* 7:391–397, 1983.

126. Hannington-Kiff, J. G. Relief of causalgia in limbs by regional intravenous guanethidine. *Br. Med. J.* 2:367–368, 1979.

127. Hannington-Kiff, J. G. Relief of Sudeck's atrophy by regional intravenous guanethidine. *Lancet* 1:1132–1133, 1977.
128. Hannington-Kiff, J. G. Intravenous regional sympathetic block with guanethidine. *Lancet* 1:1019–1020, 1974.
129. Hardy, W. G., Posch, J. L., Webster, J. E., et al. The problem of minor and major causalgias. *Am. J. Surg.* 95:545–554, 1958.
130. Harper, C. M., Low, P. A., Fealey, R. D., et al. Utility of thermography in the diagnosis of lumbosacral radiculopathy. *Neurology* 41:1010–1014, 1991.
131. Hart, G. R. and Anderson, R. J. Withdrawal syndromes and the cessation of antihypertensive therapy. *Arch. Intern. Med.* 141:1125–1127, 1981.
132. Hedberg, A. and Mattsson, H. Beta adrenoreceptor interaction of full and partial agonists in the cat heart and soleus muscle. *J. Pharmacol. Exp. Ther.* 219:798–808, 1981.
133. Helmrich, S. P., Ragland, D. R., Leung, R. W., et al. Physical activity and reduced occurrence of non-insulin-dependent diabetes mellitus. *N. Engl. J. Med.* 325(3):147, 1991.
134. Helms, C. A., O'Brien, E. G., and Katzberg, R. W. Segmental reflex sympathetic dystrophy syndrome. *Radiology* 35:67, 1980.
135. Hendler, M., Uematesu, S., et al. Thermographic validation of physical complaints of "psychogenic pain" patients. *Psychosomatics* 23:283, 1982.
136. Hobelmann, C. F. and Dellon, A. L. Use of prolonged sympathetic blockade as an adjunct to surgery in the patient with sympathetic maintained pain. *Microsurgery* 10:151–153, 1989.
137. Hodges, D. and McGuire, T. J. Burning and pain after injury — Is it causalgia or reflex sympathetic dystrophy?. *Postgrad. Med.* 83(2):185, 1988.
138. Hoffert, M. J., Greenberg, R. P., Wolskee, P. J., et al. Abnormal and collateral innervations of sympathetic and peripheral sensory fields associated with a case of causalgia. *Pain* 20:1–12, 1984.
139. Hokfelt, T., Elfvin, L.-G., Schultzgerg, M., et al. On the occurrence of substance P-containing fibers in sympathetic ganglia: Immunohistochemical evidence. *Brain Res.* 132:29–41, 1977.
140. Hokfelt, T., Johannsson, O., Fuxe, K., Goldstein, M., and Park, D. Immunohistochemical studies on the localization and distribution of monoamine neuron systems in the rat brain. l. Tyrosine hydroxylase in the mesencephalon and diencephalon. *Med. Biol.* 54:427–453, 1976.
141. Hokfelt, T., Kellerth, J.-O., Nilsson, G., and Pernow, B. Substance P: Localization in the central nervous system and in some primary sensory neurons. *Science* 190:889–890, 1975.
142. Hokfelt, T., Kellerth, J.-O., Nilsson, G., and Pernow, B. Experimental immunohistochemical studies on the localization and distribution of substance P in cat primary sensory neurons. *Brain Res.* 100:235–252, 1975.
143. Holder, L. E. and MacKinnon, S. E. Reflex sympathetic dystrophy in the hands: Clinical and scintigraphic criteria. *Radiology* 152:517, 1984.
144. Holland, A. J. C., Davies, D. H., and Wallace, D. H. Sympathetic blockade of isolated limbs by intravenous guanethidine. *Can. Anaesth. Soc. J.* 24:597, 1977.
145. Holmberg, E. and Waldeck, B. Analysis of the B-receptor mediated effects of fast-contracting skeletal muscle in vitro. *Naunyn Schmiedebergs Arch. Pharmacol.* 303:109–113, 1977.
146. Homans, J. Minor causalgia: A hyperesthetic neurovascular syndrome. *N. Engl. J. Med.* 222:870–874, 1940.
147. Hooshmand, H., Radfar, R., and Beckner, E. The neurophysiological aspects of electrical injuries. *Clin. EEG* 20(111):11–19, 1989.
148. Hooshmand, H., Radfar, F., and Beckner, E. The technical and clinical aspects of topographic brain mapping. *Clin. EEG* 20(4):2 1989.
149. Hooshmand, H., Director, K., Beckner, E., and Radfar, F. Topographic brain mapping in head injuries. *J. Clin. Neurophysiol.* 4:228–229, 1987.
150. Hooshmand, H. and Radfar, F. IV ACTH as an adjunct in narcotic detoxification. *Neurology* 37(Suppl. 1):239, 1987.
151. Hooshmand, H., Director, K., Beckner, E., and Radfar, F. Technical aspects of topographic brain mapping. *J. Clin. Neurophysiol.* 4(3):226–227, 1987.
152. Horowitz, S. H. Iatrogenic causalgia: Classification, clinical findings, and legal ramifications. *Arch. Neurol.* 41:821–824, 1984.
153. Howe, J. F., Loeser, J. D., and Calvin, W. H. Mechanosensitivity of dorsal root ganglia and chronically injured axons: A physiological basis for the radicular pain of nerve root compression. *Pain* 3:25–41, 1977.
154. Hubbard, J. E. Statistical review of thermography in a neurology practice, pain evaluation. *Postgrad. Med.* Special Edition 65–72, 1986.
155. Hubbard, J. E. Statistical review of thermography in a neurology practice. Proceedings of the First Annual Meeting of the Academy of Neuro-Muscular Thermography, May 1985. *Postgrad. Med.* Special Edition March 1986.
156. Hunter, C. Myalgia of the abdominal wall. *Can. Med. Assoc. J.* 28:157–161, 1933.
157. Huskinson, E. C. Visual analog scale. Melzack, R. ed. In *Pain Measurement and Assessment*. Raven Press. New York, 1983, pp. 33–37.

158. Hypothalamic Regulation of Endocrine Functions. Stuttgart Schattauer 1975, WL312S989S 1973. Prolactin Secretion in Humans: 379–409.

159. Intenzo, C. and Kim, S. Scintigraphic patterns of the reflex sympathetic dystrophy syndrome of the lower extremities. *Clin. Nuclear Med.* 14:657, 1989.

160. Jacobowitz, D. M. and O'Donohue, T. L. a-Melanocyte stimulating hormone: Immunohistochemical identification and mapping in neurons of rat brain. *Proc. Natl. Acad. Sci. U.S.A.* 75:6300–6304, 1978.

161. Jaffe, C. C. Why an image? *Invest. Radiol.* 19:248–249, 1984.

162. Janig, W. Causalgia and reflex sympathetic dystrophy: In which way is the sympathetic nervous system involved? *Trends Neurosci.* 471–477, 1985.

163. Jankovic, J. and VanDerLinder, C. Dystonia and tremor induced by peripheral trauma: Predisposing factors. *J. Neurol. Neurosurg. Psychiat.* 51:1512–1519, 1988.

164. Jennes, L. and Stumpf, W. E. LHRH-systems in the brain of the golden hamster. *Cell Tissue Res.* 290:239–256, 1980.

165. Kalaska, J. and Pomeranz, B. Chronic peripheral nerve injuries after the somatotopic organization of the cuneate nucleus in kittens. *Brain Res.* 236:35–47, 1982.

166. Kawano, M., Matsuoka, M., et al. Autogenic training as an effective treatment for reflex neurovascular dystrophy: A case report. *Acta Paediatr. Jpn.* 31:500–503, 1989.

167. Keegan, J. J. and Garrett, F. D. The segmental distribution of the cutaneous nerves in the limbs of man. *Anat. Rec.* 102:409–437, 1948.

168. Kenins, P. Identification of the unmyelinated sensory nerves which evoke plasma extravasation in response to autonomic stimulation. *Neurosci. Lett.* 25:137–141, 1981.

169. Kesler, R. W., Saulsbury, F. T., et al. Reflex sympathetic dystrophy in children: Treatment with transcutaneous electric nerve stimulation. *Pediatrics* 82(5):728, 1988.

170. Kirklin, J. W., Henoweth, A. I., et al. Causalgia: A review of its characteristics, diagnosis and treatment. *Surgery* 21:321, 1947.

171. Kiss, F. Sympathetic elements in cranial and spinal ganglia. *J. Anat.* 66:488–498, 1932.

172. Kleinert, H. E., Cole, N. M., Wayne, L., Harvey, R., Kutz, J. E., and Asasoy, E. Post-traumatic sympathetic dystrophy. *Orthop. Clin., N. Am.* 4:917–927, 1973.

173. Kleinman, D., Rosen, R. C., et al. Combined anesthetic and surgical treatment of reflex sympathetic dystrophy following a healed crush injury of the foot. *J. Foot Surg.* 29(1), 1990.

174. Koppers, V. B. Three-phase scintigraphy in the Sudeck syndrome: Comparison of the radiological and clinical examination. *Fortschr. Roentgenstr.* 137:564, 1982.

175. Kozin, F., et al. Bone scintigraphy in the reflex sympathetic dystrophy syndrome. *Radiology* 138:437, 1981.

176. Kozin, F., McCarty, D. J., Sims, J., and Genant, H. The reflex sympathetic dystrophy syndrome. *J. Clin. Histol. Studies.* Evidence for bilaterality, response to corticosteroids and articular involvement. *Am. J. Med.* 60:321–331, 1976.

177. Kozin, F., Genant, H., Beckerman, C., et al. The reflex sympathetic dystrophy syndrome, II. Roentgenographic and scintigraphic evidence of bilaterality and of periarticular accentuation. *Am. J. Med.* 60:332–338, 1976.

178. Kozin, F., et al. The reflex sympathetic dystrophy syndrome (RSDS). III. Scintigraphic studies: Further evidence for the therapeutic efficacy of systemic corticosteroids and proposed diagnostic criteria. *Am. J. Med.* 70:23, 1981.

179. Kuba, K. Effects of cathecholamines on the neuromuscular junction in the rat diaphragm. *J. Physiol.* 211:551–570, 1970.

180. Kure, K., Nitta, Y., Tuzi, M., et al. Demonstration of special parasympathetic nerve fibers in the dorsal or posterior roots of the lumbar region of the spine. *Q. J. Exp. Physiol.* 18:333–344, 1928.

181. Kure, K., Saegusa, G., Kawaguchi, K., et al. On the parasympathetic (spinal parasympathetic) fibers in the dorsal roots and their cells of origin in the spinal cord. *Q. J. Exp. Physiol.* 20:51–66, 1930.

182. Ladd, A. L., DeHaven, D. E., et al. Reflex sympathetic imbalance, Response to epidural blockades. *Am. J. Sports Med.* 17(5), 1989.

183. Lance, J. W. Fifty years of migraine research. *Aust. N.Z. J. Med.* 18:311–317, 1988.

184. Lance, J. W., Lambert, G. A., Goadsby, P. J., et al. 5-Hydroxtryptamine and its putative aetiological involvement in migraine. *Cephalalgia* Suppl. 9:7–13, 1989.

185. Langlohn, N. D., et al. Transient painful osteoporosis of the lower extremities. *J. Bone Joint Surg.* 55A:1188, 1973.

186. Lankford, L. L. and Thompson, J. E. Reflex sympathetic dystrophy, upper and lower extremity: Diagnosis and managment. In *The American Academy of Orthopaedic Surgeons. Instructional Course Lectures*, Vol. 26. St. Louis: C. V. Mosby, 1977, pp. 163–178.

187. Lemahieu, R. A., VanLaere, C., et al. Reflex sympathetic dystrophy: An underreported syndrome in children? *Pediatrics* 147:47–50, 1988.

188. Lesquesne, M. Etiologie et pathologie des algodystrophyes. *Presse Med.* 76:953, 1968.

189. Leriche, R. De La Causalgie envisage come une nevrite du sympaatic et son traitment per la denudation et l'exicion des plexus nerveux periarteriels. *Presse Med.* 24:178, 1916.
190. Leriche, R. and Policard, J. *Les Problems de la Physiologie Normal et Pathologie de l'os.* Paris: Mason, 1926.
191. Lesquesne, M., et al. Partial transient osteoporosis. *Skeletal Radiol.* 2:1, 1977.
192. Lewis, T. *Pain.* New York: Macmillan, 1942.
193. Lewis, D. and Gatewood, W. Treatment of causalgia: Results of intraneural injection of 60% alcohol. *JAMA* 74:1, 1920.
194. Lichtenstein, L. *Diseases of Bone and Joints*, 2nd ed., St. Louis: C. V. Mosby, 1975, p. 244.
195. Liu-Chen L.-Y., Mayber M., and Moskowitz, M. A. Immunohistochemical evidence for a substance P-containing trigeminovascular pathway to pial arteries in cats. *Brain Res.* 168:162, 1983.
196. Livingston, W. L. *Pain Mechanisms.* New York: Plenum Press, 1976, pp. 124–125.
197. Livingston, W. K. *Pain Mechanisms: A Physiologic Interpretation of Causalgia and Its Related States.* New York: Macmillan, 1943.
198. Ljungdahl, A., Hokfeld, T., and Nilsson, G. Distribution of substance P-like immunoreeactivity in the central nervous system of the rat. I. Cell bodies and terminals. *Neuroscience* 3:861–943, 1978.
199. Lofstrom, J. D., Lloyd, J. W., and Cousins, M. J. Sympathetic neural blockade of the upper and lower extremity. In Cousins M. J., and Bridenbaugh P. O., eds. *Neural Blockade in Clinical Anesthesia and Management of Pain.* Philadelphia: J. B. Lippincott, 1980, pp. 574–575, 620–624.
200. Loh, L., Nathan, P. W., Scott, G. D., and Wilson, P. G. Effects of regional guanethidine infusion in certain painful states. *J. Neurol. Neurosurg. Psychiat.* 43:446–451, 1980.
201. Loh, L., Nathan, P. W., et al. Pain due to lesions of the central nervous system removed by sympathetic block. *Br. Med. J.* 282:1026, 1981.
202. Loh, L. and Nathan, W. Painful peripheral states and sympathetic blocks. *J. Neurol. Neurosurg. Psychiat.* 41:664–671, 1978.
203. Lovisatti, L., Mori, I., and Pistolesi, G. F. Thermographic patterns of lower limb arterial disease. *Bibl. Radiol.* 6:107–114, 1975.
204. Lundblad, L., Saria, A., Lundberg, J. M., et al. Increased vascular permeability in rat nasal mucosa induced by substance P and stimulation of capsaicin-sensitive trigeminal neurons. *Acta Otolaryngol.* 96:479–484, 1983.
205. Maciewicz, R., Bouckoms, A., and Martin, J. B. Drug therapy of neuropathic pain. *Clin. J. Pain* 1:39–49, 1985.
206. Magota, F., Olshwang, D., Elmeri, D., et al. Observations on extradural morphine analgesia in various pain conditions. *Br. J. Anesth.* 52:247–252, 1980.
207. Makao, K., Nakai, Y., et al. Substantial rise of plasma beta-endorphin levels after insulin-induced hypoglycemia in human subjects. *J. Clin. Endocrinol. Metab.* 49(6):838–841, 1979.
208. Makita, Z., et al. Advanced glycosylatin end products in patients with diabetic nephropathy. *N. Engl. J. Med.* 325(12):836–842, 1991.
209. Mandel, S. and Rothrock, R. W. Sympathetic dystrophies, recognizing and managing a puzzling group of syndromes. *Postgrad. Med.* 87(8), 1990.
210. Marchettini, P., Lacerenza, M., et al. Sensitized nociceptors in reflex sympathetic dystrophies. *Funct. Neurol.* 4(2):135, 1989.
211. Marsden, C. D., Obeso, J. A., Traum, M. M., et al. Muscle spasms associated with Sudeck's atrophy after injury. *Br. Med. J.* 288:173–176, 1984.
212. Massell, T. B. Causalgic form of postphlebitic syndrome — A variety of reflex sympathetic dystrophy caused by acute deep thrombophlebitis. *West. J. Med.* 149:3, 1988.
213. Mayer, D. J., Price, D. D., and Becer, D. R. Neurophysiology of the anterolateral spinal cord neurons contributing to pain perception in man. *Pain* 1:51–58, 1973.
214. Mayfield, F. H., Devine, and J. W. Causalgia. *Surg. Gynecol. Obstet.* 80:631, 1945.
215. Mayfield, F. H. *Causalgia.* Springfield, IL: Charles C Thomas, 1951.
216. McCulloch, J., Uddman, R., Kingman, T., et al. Calcitonin gene-related polypeptide: Functional role in cerebrovascular regulation. *Proc Natl. Acad. Sci. U.S.A.* 83:5731, 1986.
217. McLachlan, E. M. and Tanig, W. The cell bodies of origin of sympathetic and sensory axons in some skin and muscle nerves of the cat hindlimb. *J. Comp. Neurol.* 214:115–130, 1983.
218. McNeil, G. N., Shaw, P. K., et al. Substitution of alcohol for propranolol in a case of propranolol related depression. *Am. J. Psychiat.* 130:1187–1188, 1982.
219. Melzack, R. The McGill Pain Questionnaire: Major properties and scoring methods. *Pain.* 1:277–299, 1975.
220. Melzack, R. and Wall, P. D. Pain mechanisms. A new theory. *Science* 150:971–979, 1965.
221. Melzack, R. Phantom limb pain. *Anesthesiology* 35:404, 1971.
222. Meredith, I. T., Broughton, A., Jennings, G. L., et al. Evidence of a selective increase in cardiac sympathetic activity in patients with sustained ventricular arrhythmias. *N. Engl. J. Med.* 325(9):618, 1991.

223. Mersky, H., Albe-Fessard, D. G., Bonica, J. J., et al. Pain terms: A list with definitions and notes on usage. *Pain* 6:249–252, 1979.

224. Meyer, R. A., Raja, S., and Campbell, J. N. Coupling of action potential activity between unmyelinated fibers in the peripheral nerve of money. *Science* 227:184–186, 1985.

224a. Meyer, R. A., Raja, S. N., Campbell, J. N., et al. Neural activity originating from a neuroma in the baboon. *Brain Res.* 325:255–260, 1985.

225. Meyer, E., Ferguson, S., Zatorre, R. J., et al. Attention modulator somatosensory cerebral blood flow response to vibrotactile stimulation as measured by positive emissions tomography. *Ann. Neurol.* 29(4):440–443, 1991.

226. Miller, D. S. and DeTakats, G. Postraumatic dystrophy of the extremities. Sudeck's atrophy. *Surg. Gynecol. Obstet.* 75:558–582, 1942.

227. Miller, R. D., Munger, W. L., and Powell, P. E. Chronic pain and local anesthetic neural blockade. Cousins, J. J., and Bridenbaugh, P. E., eds. In *Neural Blockade in Clinical Anesthesia and Management of Pain.* Philadelphia: J. B. Lippincott 1980, pp. 616–636.

228. Mitchell, S. W. Injuries of Nerves and Their Consequences. New York: Dover, 1877, pp. 363–368.

229. Mitchell, GAG. *Anatomy of the Autonomic Nervous System.* London: Livingston, 1955.

230. Mitchell, S. W. *Injuries of Nerves and Their Consequences.* London, Smith Elder, 1872.

231. Montgomery, I., Osward, I., Morgan, K., et al. Trazodone enhances sleep in subjective quality but not in objective duration. *Br. J. Clin. Pharmacol.* 16:139–144, 1983.

232. Morton, M. J. and Pitel, M. L. Reflex sympathetic dystrophy syndrome complicating the management of TMJ symptoms. A case report. *J. Craniomand. Pract.* 7(3):239–242, 1989.

233. Moskowitz, M. A. Basic mechanisms in vascular headache. *Neorol. Clin. N.A.* 801–815, 1990.

234. Moskowitz, M. A., Reinhard, J. F., Jr., Romero, J., et al. Neurotransmitters and the fifth cranial nerve; is there a relation to the headache phase of migraine. *Lancet.* 2:883–885, 1979.

235. Moskowitz, M. A. The visceral organ brain. *Neurology* 41:182–186, 1991.

236. Moskowitz, M. A. The neurobiology of vascular head pain. *Ann. Neurol.* 16:157–168, 1984.

237. Mountcastle, V. B. *Medical Physiology,* 13th ed. St. Louis: C.V. Mosby, 1974.

238. Mouret, J., Lemoine, P., Minuitt, M. P., et al. Effects of trazodone on the sleep of depressed subjects: A polygraphic study. *Psychopharmacology* 95:S37-S43, 1988.

239. Muratorio, A., Maggini, C., Coccagna, G., et al. Polygraphic study of the all-night sleep pattern in neurotic and depressed patients treated with trazodone. Ban T. A. and Silvestrini, B., eds. In *Trazodone, Modern Problems in Pharmacopsychiatry,* Vol. 9. Basel, Switzerland: S. Karger, 1947, pp. 182–189.

240. Myers, G. A. and Fields, H. L. Causalgia treated by selective large fiber stimulation of peripheral nerve. *Brain* 95:163, 1972.

241. Nashold, H. S. Dorsal root entry zone lesions: Status in 1984. *Neurosurgery* 15:942–944, 1984.

242. Nathan, P. W. On the pathogenesis of causalgia in peripheral nerve injuries. *Brain* 70:145, 1947.

243. Nedjar, C. and Ficat, C. Interet de la reserpine intraveineuse dans le traitement de l'algodystrophie reflexe. *Aggressologie* 7:317–320, 1982.

244. Nemeroff, C. B. Psychoneuroendocrinology in psychiatry. *J. Clin. Psychiat.* 50(5) (Suppl.):15–16, 1989.

245. Nielsen, V. K. Pathophysiology of hemifacial spasm: II. Lateral spread of the supraorbital nerve reflex. *Neurology* 34:427–431, 1984.

246. Nielsen, V. K. Pathophysiology of hemifacial spasm: I. Ephaptic transmission and ectopic excitations. *Neurology* 34:418–431, 1984.

247. Nielson, V. K., and Jannetta, P. J. Pathophysiology of hemifacial spasm: III. Effects of facial nerve decompression. *Neurology* 34:891–897, 1984.

248. Nies, A. S. In *Clinical Pharmacology: Basic Principles in Therapeutics.* Melmon, K. L. and Morelli, H. F., eds. New York: Macmillan, 1972.

249. Ochoa, J. The newly recognized painful ABC syndrome! Thermographic aspects. *Thermology* 2:65, 1986.

250. Ochoa, J. Techniques in assessing peripheral nervous system function. *Am J. EEG Technol.* 30:29–44, 1990.

251. Ochoa, J. L. and Torebjork, E. K. Pain from skin and muscle. *Pain* (Suppl.), 1:587, 1981.

252. Ochoa, J. L. and Torebjork, H. E. Sensations evoked by intraneural microstimulation of single mechano-receptor units innervating the human hand. *J. Physiol. (London)* 342:633–654, 1983.

253. Odderson, I. R. and Czerniecki, J. M. Reflex sympathetic dystrophy in an amputee: Case study. *Arch. Phys. Med. Rehabil.* 71:161–163, 1990.

254. Olesen, J. Effect of serotonin on regional cerebral blood flow (rCBF) in man. *Cephalalgia* 1:7–10, 1981.

255. Olesen, J. The ischemic hypotheses of migraine. *Arch. Neurol.* 44:321–322, 1987.

256. Olesen, J., Larsen, B., and Lauritzen, M. Focal hyperemia followed by spreading oligemia and impaired activation of rCBF in classic migraine. *Ann. Neurol.* 9:344–352, 1981.

257. Olesen, J., Telt-Hansen, P., Henriksen, L., et al. The common migraine attack may not be initiated by cerebral ischemia. *Lancet* 2:438–440, 1981.

258. Omer, G. and Thomas, S. Treatment of causalgia: A review of cases at Brooke General Hospital. *Texas Med.* 67:93, 1971.

259. Orbeli, L. A. Die sympathtische Innervation der Skelettmuskeln. *Izv. Petrog. Nauch. Inst. P. F. Lesyafta.* 187–197, 1923.

260. Osada, E., Sakaya, S., and Seri, K. Pharmacological studies of mabuterol, a new selective B2-stimulant. *Arzneimittelforschung* 34:1652–1658, 1984.

261. Ostergren, I. R., Fagrell, B., and Stranden, E. Skin microvascular circulation in the sympathetic dystrophies evaluated by videophotometric capillaroscopy and laser Doppler fluxmetry. *Eur. J. Clin. Invest.* 18:305–308, 1988.

262. Parry, C. B. Pain in avulsion lesions of the brachial plexus. *Neurosurgery* 9(1):41–53, 1980.

263. Parry, C. W. Management of pain in avulsion lesions of the brachial plexus. Bonica, J. J., Lindblom, U., and Iggo, A., eds. In *Proceedings of the Third World Congress on Pain.* New York: Raven Press, 1983, pp. 751–761. (*Adv. Pain Res. Ther.* Vol. 5).

264. Passariello, R., Masciocchi, C., Quarta Colosso, L., et al. Reflex sympathetic dystrophy syndrome. *Rays* 14:4, 1989.

265. Patman, R. D., Thompson, J. E., and Persson, A. V. Management of posttraumatic pain syndromes: A report of 113 cases. *Ann. Surg.* 177:780–787, 1973.

266. Patten, S. B. Propranolol and depression: Evidence from the antihypertensive trials. *Can. J. Psychiat.* 35:257–258, 1990.

267. Patterson, J. R. Psychosis following discontinuation of a long-acting propranolol preparation. *J. Clin. Psychopharmacol.* 5:125–126, 1985.

268. Paykel, E. D., Fleminger, R., et al. Psychiatric side effects of antihypertensive drugs other than reserpine. *J. Clin. Psychopharmacol.* 2:14–39, 1982.

269. Payne, R. Neuropathic pain syndromes with special reference to causalgia and reflex sympathetic dystrophy. *Clin. J. Pain* 21(1):59–73, 1986.

270. Pelletier, G. and LeClerk, R. Immunohistochemical localization of adrenocorticotrophin in the rat brain. *Endocrine Soc.* 104:1426–1433, 1979.

271. Pelletier, G., Steinbusch, H. W. M., and Verhofstad, A. A. J. Immunoreactive substance P and serotonin are contained in the same dense core vesicles. *Nature (London)* 293:71–71, 1981.

272. Perelman, R. B., Adler, D. and Humphreys, M. Comparison of lumbosacral thermograms with CT scans. Abernathy, M., and Uematsu, S., eds. In *Medical Thermography.* Washington, D. C.: American Academy of Thermology, 1986, pp. 127–133.

273. Perelman, R. B., Wexler, C. E., Meyers, P. H., et al. Liquid crystal thermography of the spine and extremities. Its value in the diagnosis of spinal root syndromes. *J. Neurosurg.* 56:386–395, 1982.

274. Pettigrew, J. D. and Kasamatsu, T. Local perfusion of noradrenaline maintains visual cortical plasticity. *Nature (London)* 271:761–763, 1978.

275. Ghostine, S. Y., et al. Phenoxybenzamine in treatment of causalgia. *J. Neurosurg.* 60:1263, 1984.

276. Pleet, A. B., Tahmous, A. J., and Jennings, J. R. Causalgia: treatment with propranolol. *Neurology* 26:375, 1976.

277. Poehling, G. G., Pollock, F. E., et al. Reflex sympathetic dystrophy of the knee after sensory nerve injury, anthroscopy. *J. Anthroscop. Related Surg.* 4(1):31–35, 1988.

278. Pollack, M. H., Rosenbaum, J. F., et al. Propranolol and depression revisited: Three cases and a review. *J. Nerv. Ment. Dis.* 173:118–119, 1985.

279. Pollock, L. J. and Davis, L. *Peripheral Nerve Injuries.* New York: Paul B. Hoeber, 1933.

280. Poplawski, Z. J., Wiley, A. M. and Murray, J. F. Posttraumatic dystrophy of the extremities. *J. Bone Joint Surg.* 65A(5):642–653, 1983.

281. Price, J. and Mudge, A. W. A subpopulation of rat dorsal root ganglion neurons is catecholaminergic. *Nature (London)* 301:241–243, 1983.

282. Prieto, E. J., Hopson, L., Bradley, L. A., Byrne, M., Geisinger, K. F., Midax, D., and Marchisello, P. J. The language of low back pain: factor structure of the McGill Pain Questionnaire. *Pain* 8:11–19, 1980.

283. Prough, D. S., McLeskey, C. H., Boehlin, C. O., et al. Efficacy of oral nifedipine in the treatment of reflex sympathetic dystrophy. *Anesthesiology* 62:796–799, 1985.

284. Pugsley, D. J., et al. A controlled trial of labetolol, propranolol, and placebo in the management of mild to moderate hypertension. *Br. J. Clin. Pharmacol.* 7:63–68, 1979.

285. Pulst, S. M. and Haller, P. Thermographic assessment of impaired sympathetic function in peripheral nerve injuries. *J. Neurol.* 226:35–42, 1981.

286. Raskin, N. H., Levinson, S. A., Hoffman, P. M., et al. Postsympathectomy neuralgia: Amelioration with diphenylhydantoin and carbamazepine. *Am. J. Surg.* 128:75–78, 1974.

287. Raskin, N. H. *Headache,* 2nd ed. New York: Churchill Livingstone, 1988.

288. Raskin, M. M., Martinez-Lopez, M., and Sheldon, J. J. Lumbar thermography in discogenic disease. *Radiology* 119:149–152, 1976.

289. Rasminsky, M. Ectopic generation of impulses and cross talk in spinal nerve roots of "dystrophic" mice. *Ann. Neurol.* 3:351–357, 1978.

290. Rasminsky, M. Ectopic impulse generation in pathological nerve fibres. *Trends Neurosci.* 388–390, 1983.

291. Rasminsky, M. Ectopic excitation, ephaptic excitation and autoexcitation in peripheral nerve fibers of mutant mice. Culp, W. J. and Ochoa, J. L., eds. In *Abnormal Nerves and Muscles as Impulse Generators.* New York: Oxford University Press, 1982, pp. 344–362.

292. Ray, B. S. and Wolff, H. G. Experimental studies on headache: Pain-sensitive structures of the head and their sigificance in headache. *Arch. Surg.* 41:813–856, 1940.

293. Reid, et al. *J. Clin. Endocrinol. Metab.* 52:1179–1184, 1981.

294. Reiestad, F., McIlvaine, W. B., et al. Interpleural analgesia in treatment of upper extremity reflex sympathetic dystrophy. *Anesth. Analg.* 69:671–673, 1989.

295. Resminsky, M. Ephaptic transmission between single nerve fibres in the spinal nerve roots of dystrophic mice. *J. Physiol. (London)* 305:151–169, 1980.

296. Richards, R. L. Causalgia: A centennial review. *Arch. Neurol.* 16:339–350, 1967.

297. Richter, C. P. and Woodrugg, B. G. Lumbar sympathetic dermatomes in man determined by the electrical skin resistance method. *J. Neurophysiol.* 8:323–338, 1945.

298. Rizzi, R., Visentin, M. and Mazzetti, G. Reflex sympathetic dystrophy. Benedetti, C., Chapman, C. R., and Morrica, G., eds. In *Recent Advances in the Management of Pain.* New York: Raven Press, 1984, pp. 451–464 (*Adv. Pain Res.* Vol. 7).

299. Robaina, F. J., Rodriguez, J. L., et al. Transcutaneous electrical nerve stimulation and spinal cord stimulation for pain relief in reflex sympathetic dystrophy. *Stereotact. Funct. Neurosurg.* 52:53–62, 1989.

300. Robberect, W., VanHees, J., et al. Painful muscle spasms complicating algodystrophy: Central or peripheral disease? *J. Neurol. Neurosurg. Psychiat.* 51:563–567, 1988.

301. Roberts, W. J. An hypothesis on the physiological basis for causalgia and related pains. *Pain* 24:297, 1986.

302. Roberts, W. J. and Elardo, S. M. Sympathetic activation of unmyelinated mechanoreceptors in cat skin. *Brain Res.* 339:123–125, 1985.

303. Roig-Escofet, D., Rodriguez-Moreno, J. and Ruiz Martin, J. M. Concept and limits of the reflex sympathetic dystrophy. *Clin. Rheumatol.* 8 (Suppl. 2):104–108, 1989.

304. Rosen, P. S. and Graham, W. The shoulder-hand syndrome: Historical review with observation on seventy-three patients. *Can. Med. Assoc. J.* 77:86, 1975.

305. Rosenblum, J. Documentation of thermographic objectivity in pain syndromes. *Postgrad. Med.* 59, 1986.

306. Rosomoff, H. L. Do Herniated Discs Produce Pain? *Clin. J. Pain* 1:2, 1985.

307. Rothberg, J. M., Tahmoush, A. J., et al. The epidemiology of causalgia among soldiers wounded in Vietnam. *Milit. Med.* 148:347, 1983.

308. Rowlingson, J. C. The sympathetic dystrophies. *Int. Anesthesiol. Clin.* 21:117–129, 1983.

309. Ruben, J. E. Causalgia: Reflex sympathetic nerve dystrophy. *Med. Trial. Tech. Q.* 16:39–44, 1969.

310. Ruch, T. C. *Pathophysiology of pain: Medical physiology and Biophysics*, 18th ed. Philadelphia: W. B. Saunders, 1960, pp. 350–368.

311. Russeck, H. I. Shoulder-hand syndrome following myocardial infarction. *Med. Clin. N.A.* 42:1555, 1958.

312. Saidman, J. *Diagnostic et Traitement Des Maladies de la Colonne Vertebrate.* Paris: G. Doin, 1949.

313. Saito, K., Greenberg, S., and Moskowitz, M. A. Trigeminal origin of beta-prepotachykinin in feline pial blood vessels. *Neurosci. Lett.* 76:69, 1987.

314. Santini, D. M. Towards a theory of sympathetic sensory coupling; the primary neuron as a feedback target of the sympathetic termina. Otterman, Y., ed. In *Sensory Functions of the Skin in Primates with Special Reference to Man*, Vol. 27. Oxford: Pergamon Press, 1976, pp. 489–502.

315. Santo, J. L., Arias, L. M., et al. Bilateral cingulumotomy in the treatment of reflex sympathetic dystrophy, *Pain* 41:55–59, 1990.

316. Sato, A. and Schmidt, R. F. Somatosympathetic reflexes: Afferent fibers, central pathways, discharge characteristics. *Physiol. Rev.* 53:916–947, 1973.

317. Scadding, J. W. Development of ongoing activity, mechanosensitivity, and adrenalin sensitivity in severed peripheral nerve axons. *Exp. Neurol.* 73:345–364, 1981.

318. Scadding, J. W., Wall, P. D., Parry, C. B. W., and Brook, D. M. Clinical trials of propranolol in post-traumatic neuralgia. *Pain* 14:283–292, 1982.

319. Schady, W. J. L., Torebjork, H. E., and Ochoa, J. L. Cerebral localization function from the input of single mechanoreceptive units in man. *Acta Physiol. Scand.* 119:277–285, 1983.

320. Schapira, D., Barron, S. A., et al. Reflex sympathetic dystrophy syndrome coincident with acute diabetic neuropathy. *J. Rheumatol.* 15:1, 1988.

321. Scharf, M. D. and Sachais, B. A. Sleep Laboratory Evaluation of the Effects and Efficacy of Trazodone in Depressed Insomniac Patients, 1990. Bristol-Myers Squibb Company, Evansville, Indiana 47721.

322. Scherokman, B., Hussain, F., Cuetler, A., et al. Peripheral dystonia. *Arch. Neurol.* 43:830–832, 1986.

323. Schiller, J. E. Reflex sympathetic dystrophy of the foot and ankle in children and adolescents. *J. Am. Podiatr. Med. Assoc.* 79(11):545, 1989.

324. Schmidt, A. Zur Pathogie und Therapie des Muskelrheumatisimus (Myalgie). *Muench. Med. Wochenschrift* 63:593–595, 1916.

325. Schmidt, R. E., Chae, H. Y., Parvin, C. A., et al. Neuroaxonal dystrophy in aging human sympathetic ganglia. *Am. J. Pathol.* 136(6):1327–1338, 1990.

326. Schott, G. D. Mechanisms of causalgia and related clinical conditions. *Brain* 109:717–738, 1986.

327. Schott, G. D. The relationship of peripheral trauma and pain to dystonia. *J. Neurol. Neurosurg. Psychiat.* 48:698–701, 1985.

328. Schott, G. D. Induction of involuntary movements by peripheral trauma: an analogy with causalgia. *Lancet* 2:712–716, 1986.

329. Schumacker, H. B., Speigel, I. J., and Upjohn, R. H. Causalgia I. The role of sympathetic interruption in treatment. *Surg. Gynecol. Obstet.* 86:76–86, 1948.

330. Schumacker, H. B. A personal overview of causalgia and other reflex dystrophies. *Ann. Surg.* 201:278–289, 1985.

331. Schumacker, H. B., Speigel, D., and Upjohn, R. H. Causalgia II. The signs and symptoms with particular reference to vasomotor disturbances. *Surg. Gynecol. Obstet.* 86:452–460, 1948.

332. Schwartzman, R. J. and Kerrigan, J. The movement disorder of reflex sympathetic dystrophy. *Neurology* 40:57, 1990.

333. Scott, G. Clinical features of algodystrophy: Is the sympathetic nervous system involved? *Funct. Neurol.* 4(2):131, 1989.

334. Seitzer, A. and Devor, M. Ephaptic transmission in chronically damaged peripheral nerves. *Neurology* 29:1061–1064, 1979.

335. Serre, H., Simon, L., and Claustre, J. Sympathetic dystrophy of the foot. *Rev. Rheum.* 34:722–732, 1967.

336. Shih, W. J. and Pulmao, C. Hand and forearm Tc-99m HMDP bone image findings of reflex sympathetic dystrophy similar to those of radiopharmaceutical arterial administration in the arm. *Clin. Nuclear Med.* 14:298, 1989.

337. Sicuteri, F., Testi, A., and Anselmi, B. Biochemical investigations in headache: Increase in hydroxyindole acetic acid excretion during migraine attacks. *Int. Arch. Allergy Appl. Immunol.* 19:55–58, 1961.

338. Silber, T. J. Anorexia nervosa and reflex sympathetic dystrophy syndrome. *Psychosomatics* 30(l), 1989.

339. Silber, T. J. and Majd, M. Reflex sympathetic dystrophy syndrome in children and adolescents. *AJDC* 142:1325, 1988.

340. Simons, D. G. and Travell, F. G. Myofascial pain syndromes. Wall. P. D. and Melzack, R., eds. In *Textbook of Pain.* Edinburgh: Churchill Livingston, 1985, pp. 263–275.

341. Simpson, G. Propranolol for causalgia and Sudek's atrophy. *JAMA* 227:327, 1974.

342. Sims, J. and Galvin, M. R. Pediatric psychopharmocologic uses of propranolol. *JCPN* 3(1):18–24, 1990.

343. Skinner, J. E. and King, G. L. Electrogenesis of event-related slow potentials in the cerebral cortex of conscious animals. Pfurtscheller, G. and Buser, P., eds. In *Rhythmic EEG Activities and Cortical Activities.* Vol 10. New York: Elsevier North-Holland Biomedical Press, 1980, pp. 21–32.

344. Skinner, J. E. and Molnar, M. Event-related extracellular potassium ion activity changes in the frontal cortex of the conscious cat. *J. Neurophysiol.* 49:204–215, 1983.

345. Skinner, J. E., Welch, K. M. A., Reed, J. C., et al. Psychological stress reduces cyclic 3′, 5′-adenosine monophosphate level in the parietal cortex of the conscious rat. *J. Neurochem.* 30:691–698, 1978.

346. Skinner, J. E. and Yingling, C. D. Central gating mechanisms that regulate event-related potentials and behavior: A neural model for attention. Desmedt, J. E., ed. In *Progress in Clinical Neurophysiology.* Vol l. New York: S. Karger, 1977, pp. 70–96.

347. Sladek, J. R. and Sladek, C. D. Localization of serotonin within tanycytes of the rat median eminence. *Cell Tissue Res.* 186:465–474, 1978.

348. Slessor, A. J. Causalgia: A review of 22 cases. *Edinburgh Med. J.* 44:563, 1948.

349. Snider, R. M. and Gerald, M. C. Studies on the mechanism of (+)-amphetamine enhancement of neuromuscular transmission: Muscle contraction, electrophysiological and biochemical results. *J. Pharmacol. Exp. Ther.* 221:14–21, 1982.

350. Spiegel, I. J. and Milowsky, J. I. Causalgia. *JAMA* 127:9–15, 1945.

351. Spiegel, I. J. and Milowsky, J. L. Causalgia: Preliminary report of nine cases treated successfully by surgical and chemical interruption of sympathetic pathways. *JAMA* 127:9, 1945.

352. Standards of neuro-muscular thermography of the Academy of Neuro-Muscular Thermography. *Clin. Thermog. J. Acad. Neuro-Musc. Thermog.* August 1989.

353. Stary, O. The pathogenesis of discogenic disease. *Rev. Czech. Med.* 2:1–16, 1956.

354. Steinbrocker, O. The shoulder-hand syndrome, associated painful homolateral disability of the shoulder and swelling and atrophy of the hand. *Am. J. Med.* 3:402–406, 1947.

355. Stellar, S., Ahrens, S., Meibohm, A. R., et al. Migraine prevention with timolol. *JAMA* 252(18), 1984.

356. Stevens, R. T. Catecholamine varicosities in cat dorsal root ganglion and spinal ventral roots. *Brain Res.* 261:151–154, 1983.

357. Stoudemire, A., et al. Propranolol and depression: A reevaluation based on a pilot clinical trial. *Psychiatr Med.* 2:211–218, 1984.

358. Stubbs, W. A., Delitala, G., Jones, A., et al. Hormonal and metabolic responses to an enkephalin analogue in normal man. *Lancet* 2(8102):1225–1227, 1978.

359. Sudeck, P. Uber die akute entzundickle Knockenatrophie. *Arch. Klin. Chir.* 62:147, 1900.

360. Sumatriptan International Study Group: Treatment of Migraine Attacks with Sumatriptan. *N. Engl. J. Med.* 325(5):316, 1991.

361. Sumatriptan Cluster Headache Study Group: Treatment of Acute Cluster Headache with Sumatriptan. *N. Engl. J. Med.* 325(5):322, 1991.

362. Sunderland, S. and Kelly, M. The painful sequelae of injuries to peripheral nerves. *Aust. N.Z. J. Surg.* 18:75, 1948.

363. Sunderland, S. *Nerves and Nerve Injuries.* Edinburgh: Churchill Livington, 1968.

364. Sweet, W. H. and Poletti, C. E. Causalgia and sympathetic dystrophy (Sudeck's atrophy). Aronoff, G. M., ed. In *Evaluation and Treatment of Chronic Pain.* Baltimore: Urban and Scharzenberg, 1985, pp. 149–165.

365. Swerdlow, M. Anticonvulsant drugs and chronic pain. *Clin. Neuropharmacol.* 7:51–82, 1984.

366. Tabira, T., Shibasaki, H., and Kuroiwa, Y. Reflex sympathetic dystrophy (causalgia) treatment with guanethidine. *Arch. Neurol.* 40:430–432, 1983.

367. Tahmoush, A. J. Causalgia: Redefinition as a clinical pain syndrome. *Pain* 10(2):187–197, 1981.

368. Thomas, D. G. T. and Jones, T. J. Dorsal root entry lesions (Nashold's procedure) in brachial plexus avulsion. *Neurosurgery* 13:966–968, 1984.

369. Thompson, J. E. The diagnosis and managment of posttraumatic pain syndromes (causalgia). *Aust. N.Z. J. Surg.* 49:299–304, 1979.

370. Thompson, J. E., Patman, D., and Persson, A. V. Management of post-traumatic pain syndromes (causalgia). *Am. Surg.* 41:599–602, 1975.

371. Tieges, O. W. Innervation of voluntary muscle. *Physiol. Rev.* 33:90–144, 1953.

372. Tooke, J. E., Ostergren, J., and Fagrell, B. Synchronous assessment of human skin microcirculation by laser Doppler flowmetry and dynamic capillaroscopy. *Int. J. Microcirc.* 2:277–284, 1983.

373. Torebjork, H. E. and Ochoa, J. L. Specific sensations evoked by activity in single identified sensory units in man. *Acta Physiol. Scand.* 110:445–447, 1980.

374. Torebjork, H. E., Ochoa, J. L., and Schady, W. Referred pain from intraneural stimulation of muscle fascicles in the median nerve. *Pain* 18:145–156, 1984.

375. Tracy, D. G. and Cockett, F. B. Pain in the lower limb after sympathectomy. *Lancet* 1:12–14, 1957.

376. Travell, J. Myofascial trigger points: Clinical view. Bonica, J. J. and Albe-Fessard, D., eds. In *Advances in Pain Research and Therapy*, Vol. 1. New York: Raven Press, 1976, pp. 919–926.

377. Travell, J. Myofascial trigger points: Clinical view. Bonica, J. J. and Albe-Fessard, D., eds. In *Recent Advances in the Management of Pain.* New York: Raven Press, 1976, pp. 91–126 (*Adv. Pain Res. Ther.* Vol. 7).

378. Turf, R. M. and Carcardi, B. E. Causalgia: Clarifications in terminology and a case presentation. *J. Foot Surg.* 25:284–295, 1986.

379. Uematsu, S. Computerized infrared thermographic imaging in evaluation of disorders in the peripheral and central nervous system. Youmans, J. R., ed. In *Neurologic Surgery*, 3rd ed. Philadelphia: W. B. Saunders, 1990.

380. Uematsu, S. Thermographic imaging of cutaneous sensory segment on patient with peripheral nerve injury. *J. Neurosurg.* 62:716–720, 1985.

381. Uematsu, S., et al., Quantification of thermal asymmetry, Part I: Normal values and reproducibility. *J. Neurosurg.* 69:552–555, 1988.

382. Uematsu, S., Hendler, U., Hungerford, et al. Thermography and electromyography in the differential diagnosis of chronic pain syndromes and reflex sympathetic dystrophy. *Electro. Clin. Neurophysiol.* 21:164–182, 1981.

383. Ulmer, J. L. and Mayfield, F. H. Causalgia: A study of 75 cases. *Surg. Gynecol. Obstet.* 83:789, 1946.

384. Uricchio, J. and Walboroei, C. Blinded Reading of Electronic Thermography. Academy of Neuro-muscular Thermography, First Annual Meeting, May. *Postgrad. Med.* Special Edition, 47–53, 1985.

385. Valbo, A. B., Hagbarth, K. E., Torebjork, H. E., and Wallin, B. G. Somatosensory proprioceptive and sympathetic activity in human peripheral nerves. *Physiol. Rev.* 59:919–957, 1979.

386. Van Buren, J. and Kleinknecht, R. A. An evaluation of the McGill Pain Questionnaire for use in dental pain assessment, *Pain* 6:23–33, 1979.

387. Vanderhoop et al. Prevention of cisplastin neurotoxicity. *N. Engl. J. Med.* 89–94, 1990.

388. Van Der Korst, J. K., Colenbrauder, H., and Cats, A. Phenobarbital and the shoulder-hand syndrome. *Ann. Rheum. Dis.* 25:553, 1966.

389. Verrill, P. Sympathetic ganglion lesions. Wall, P. D. and Melzack, R., eds. In *Textbook of Pain.* Edinburgh: Churchill Livingstone.

390. Veterans Administration Collaborative Study Group, Comparison of propranolol and hydrochlorothiazide for the initial treatment of hypertension. II. Results of long term therapy. *JAMA* 248:2004–2011, 1982.

391. Viannikas, C., Shahani, B. T., and Young, R. R. Short-latency somatosensory-evoked potentials from radial, median, ulnar, and peroneal nerve stimulation in the assessment of cervical spondylosis. *Arch. Neurol.* 43, 1986.

392. Volkmann, R. Cited in Landoff, G.-A. Experimentelle Untersuchungen uber die "Knochenatrophie" infolge einer Immobilisation and einer akuten Arthritis. *Acta Chir. Scand.* Suppl. 71, 1942.

393. Wall, P. D. Wall, P. D. and Melzack, R. eds. In *Textbook of Pain*, 2nd ed. Edinburgh: Churchill Livingston, 1984, 2–15.

394. Wall, P. D. and Devor, M. Consequences of peripheral nerve damage in the spinal cord and in neighboring intact peripheral nerves. Ochoa, J. and Culp, W., eds. In *Abnormal Nerves and Muscles and Impulse Generators*. Oxford: Oxford University Press, 1982, pp. 589–603.

395. Wall, P. D. and Gotnick, M. Ongoing activity in peripheral nerves: The physiology and pharmacology of impulses originating from a neuroma. *Exp. Neurol.* 43:580–593, 1974.

396. Wall, J. T., Kass, J. H., Sur, M., et al. Functional reorganization in somatosensory cortical areas 3b and 7 of adult monkeys after median nerve repair: Possible relationships to sensory recovery in humans. *J. Neurosci.* 6:218–233, 1986.

397. Wallin, Torebjor, E., and Hallin, R. Preliminary observations on the pathophysiology of hyperagenia in the ausalgic pain syndrome. Zotterman, Y, ed. In *Sensory Function of the Skin in Primates*. Oxford: Pergamon, 1976, pp. 489–499.

398. Wang, J. K., Erickson, R. P., et al. Repeated stellate ganglion blocks for upper extremity reflex sympathetic dystrophy. *Regional Anesth.* 10:125, 1985.

399. Wang, J. K., Johnson, K. A., and Illstrup, D. M. Sympathetic blocks for reflex sympathetic dystrophy. *Pain* 23:13–17, 1985.

400. Watson, S. J., Richard, C. W., and Barchas, J. D. Adrenocorticotropin in rat brain: Immunocytochemical localization in cells and axons. *Science* 200:1180–1182, 1978.

401. Weir, S. *Injuries of Nerves and Their Consequences*. London: Smith Elder, 1872.

402. Welch, K. M. A. Migraine: A biobehavioral disorder. *Arch. Neurol.* 44:323–327, 1987.

403. Welch, K. M. A., Helpert, J. A., Ewing, J. R., et al. Biochemical effects of cerebral ischemia: Relevance to migraine. *Cephalalgia* 2:35–42, 1985.

404. Werman, R. and Wislicki, L. Propranolol, a curariform and cholinomimetic agent at the frog neuromuscular junction. *Comp. Gen. Pharmacol.* 2:69–81, 1971.

405. Werner, N. The role of cyclic nucleotides in the regulation of neurotransmitter release from adrenergic neurons by neuromodulator. Youdim, M. B. H., Lovenberg, W., Sarman, D. F., and Lagnado, J. R., eds. In *Essays in Neurochemistry and Neuropharmacoloy*, Vol. 4. New York: John Wiley, 1980, pp. 69–124.

406. Werner, R. and Davidoff, G. Factors affecting the sensitivity and specificity of the three-phase technetium bone scan in the diagnosis of reflex sympathetic dystrophy syndrome in the upper extremity. *J. Hand Surg.* 14A(3):520, 1989.

407. Wexler, C. E. Thermographic evaluation of trauma (spine). *Acta Thermograph.* 5:3–10, 1980.

408. Wexler, C. E. *An Overview of Liquid Crystal and Electronic Lumbar, Thoracic and Cervical Thermography*. Tarzana, CA: Thermographic Services, Inc., 1981.

409. Wexler, C. E. Diagnosis of spinal pain problems with thermography. *Diagnostic Imaging* 50, 1981.

410. Wexler, C. E, and Chafetz, N. Cervical, thoracic and lumbar thermography in the evaluation of symptomatic workers compensation patients — a blinded study. Modern Medicine, Special Supplement; Academy of Neuro-Muscular Thermography. Clinical Proceedings 53–57, September 1987.

411. White, J. C., et al. Causalgia following gunshot injuries of nerves. *Ann. Surg.* 128:161, 1948.

412. White, F. P. and Rutherford, R. B. A civilian experience with causalgia. *Arch. Surg.* 100:633, 1970.

413. White, J. C. and Sweet, W. H. *Pain and the Neurosurgeon*. Springfield, IL. Charles C Thomas, 1969.

414. Wiertz-Hoessels, E. L. Influence of trophic disturbances on skeletal muscle innervation. *Nature (London)* 204:540–542, 1964.

415. Wiesei, S. W., et al. A study of computer assisted tomography. The incidence of positive CAT scans in an asymptomatic group of patients. *Spine* 9:549–551, 1984.

416. Wilkinson, H. A. Radio frequency percutaneous upper-thoracic sympathectomy: Technique and review of indications. *N. Engl. J. Med.* 311:34–35, 1984.

417. Wilkinson, H. A. Percutaneous radiofrequency upper thoracic sympathectomy: A new technique. *Neurosurgery* 15:811–814, 1984.

418. Willis, W. D. Neurophysiology of nociception and pain in the spinal cord. Bonica, J. J., ed. In *Pain*. New York: Raven Press, 1980, pp. 77–92.

419. Wirth, F. P. and Rutherford, R. B. A civilian experience with causalgia. *Arch. Surg.* 100:633, 1970.

420. Wislicki, L. and Rosenblum, I. The effects of propranolol on normal and denervated muscle. *Arch. Int. Pharmacodyn. Ther.* 170:117–123, 1967.

421. Withrington, R. H. and Parry, W. C. B. Management of painful peripheral nerve disorders. *Br. J. Hand. Surg.* 9-B:24–28, 1984.

422. Wolff, H. G. *Headache and Other Head Pain.* New York: Oxford University Press, 1972.

423. Wood, P. D., Stefanick, M. I., Williams, P. T., and Haskell, W. L. The effects on plasma lipoproteins of a prudent weight-reducing diet, with or without exercise, in overweight men and women. *N. Engl. J. Med.* 325(7):461–466, 1991.

424. Wynn Parry, C. B. Pain in avulsion lesions of the brachial plexus. *Pain* 9:41–53, 1980.

425. Yokota, T., Furukawa, T., and Tsukagoshi, H. Motor paresis improved by sympathetic block a motor form of reflex sympathetic dystrophy? *Arch. Neurol.* 46:683–687, 1989.

426. Zucchini, M., Alberti, G., et al. Algodystrophy and related psychological features. *Funct. Neurol.* 4(2):153, 1989.

427a. Bernard, C. Recherches Experimentales sur la grand sympathique et specialement sur l'influence que le section de Ce nerf exerce sur la Chaleur animal. *C. R. Soc. Biol.* 5(2):277, 1853.

427b. Bernard, C. *Lecons sur les phenomenes de la vie.* Paris: Bailliere, 1878.

428. Hobbins, W. B. Thermography in Sports Medicine. Appenzeller, O., ed. In *Sport Medicine: Training, Fitness, Injuries.* Baltimore: Urban and Schwarzenberg, 1988, pp. 395–402.

429. Cohen, H. The mechanism of visceral pain. *Trans. Med. Soc.* 64:35, 1944.

430. Cohen, H. and Jones, H. W. The reference of cardiac pain to a phantom left arm. *Br. Heart J.* 5:67–71, 1943.

431. Hertz, A. F. The gaulstonian Lectures on the Sensibility of the Alimentary Canal in health and disease. *Lancet* 1:1051–1056;1119–1124, 1187–1193, 1911.

432. Lennander, K. G. Uber die Sensibilitate der Ansthesie bei Bruch- und Bauchoperationeer. *Bl. Chir.* 28:209–223, 1901.

433. Lewis, T. Experiments relating to peripheral mechanism involved in spasmodic arrest of circulation in fingers. A variety of Raynaud's disease. *Heart* 15:267–275, 1933.

434. Moore, R. M. and Singleton, J. A. O. Studies on the pain sensibility of arteries. *Am. J. Physiol.* 104:267–275, 1933.

435. Sterling, P. Research note. Referred cutaneous senation. *Exp. Neurol.* 41:451–456, 1973.

436. Sutton, D. C. and Lenth, H. C. Pain. *Arch. Int. Med.* 45:827–867, 1930.

437. Theobald, G. W. The role of the cerebral cortex in the appreciation of pain. *Lancet* 2:41–77, 94–96, 1949.

438. White, J. C. and Sweet, W. H. *Pain, Its Mechanisms and Neurosurgical Control.* Springfield, IL: Charles C Thomas, 1955.

439. Kelly, D. Psychosurgery and the limbic system. *Postgrad. Med. J.* 49:825–833, 1973.

440. Nauta, W. J. H. The problem of the frontal lobe, a reinterpretation. *J. Psychiat. Res.* 8, 1971.

441. Appenzeller, O. *The Autonomic Nervous System: An Introduction to Basic and Clinical Concepts,* 4th rev., Elsevier, 1990, p. 148.

442. Korner, P. E. and Uther, J. B. Reflex autonomic control of heart rate and peripheral blood flow. *Brain Res.* 87:293–303, 1975.

443. Kaada, B. Stimulation and regional activation of the amygdaloid complex with reference to functional representations. In Elexthema, B. E., ed. *The Neurobiology of the Amygdala.* New York: Plenum Press, 1972.

444. Jackson, J. H. Clinical and physiological researches on the nervous system: 1. On the anatomical and physiological localization of movements in the brain. In *Selected Writings of Hughling Jackson.* London: Hodder and Stoughton, 1931–1932.

445. Chapman, W. P., Livingston, K. E., and Poppen, J. L. Effect upon blood pressure of electrical stimulation of tips of temporal lobes in man. *J. Neurophysiol.* 13:65–71, 1950.

446. Livingston, R. B., Chapman, W. P., Livingston, K. E., and Kranitz, L. Stimulation of orbital surface of man prior to frontal lobotomy. *Res. Pub. Assoc. Res. Ment. Dis.* 27:421–432, 1948.

447. Kuhn, D. M., Wolf, W. A., et al. Reviews of the role of the central serotoninergic neuronal system in blood pressure regulation. *Hypertension* 2:243–255, 1980.

448. Sewall, H. and Sanford, E. Plethsymographic studies of the human vasomotor mechanism when exited by electrical stimulation. *J. Physiol. (London)* 179–207, 1890.

449. Pickering, G. W. and Hess, W. Vasodilation in the hands and feet in response to warming the body. *Clin. Sci.* 213–223, 1933.

450. Gibbon, J. H. and Landis, E. M. Vasodilation in the lower extremities in response to immersing the forearms in warm water. *J. Clin. Invest.* II:1019–1036, 1932.

451. Cranston, W. I. Temperature regulation. *Br. Med. J.* 2:69–75, 1966.

452. Pickering, G. W. Regulation of body temperature in health and disease. *Lancet* 1–9, 1958.

453. Appenzeller, O. The neurogenic controls of vasomotor function in the hand: A study of patients with lesions at various levels of the nervous system. Thesis, London, 1963.

454. Santorio, S. Rule of Health, Lectures on the History of Physiology during the 16th, 17th, and 18th Centuries. Cambridge, 1901.

455. Meyer, G., McElhany, M., Martin, W., and McGraw, C. P. Stereotactic cingulotomy. Laitimer and Livingston, eds. In *Surgical Approaches in Psychiatry*. Lancaster: Medical and Technical Publishing Co., 1973.

456. Bonica, J. J. The Management of Pain, Vol. 2, 2nd ed. Philadelphia: Lea & Febiger, 1990.

457. Nauta, W. J. H. Connections of the frontal lobe with the limbic system. Laitimer and Livingston, eds. In *Surgical Approaches in Psychiatry*. Lancaster: Medical and Technical Publishing Co., 1973.

458. Kelly, D. Physiological Changes during Operations on the Limbic System. *Conditional Reflex* 7:127, 1972.

459. White, J. C. and Sweet, W. H. *Pain and the Neurosurgeon*. Springfield, IL: Charles C Thomas, 1969.

460. Buerger, R. and Smith, R. Transaxillary sympathectomy (T2 to T4) for relief of vasospastic sympathetic pain of upper extremities. *Surgery* 89:764–769, 1981.

461. Sunderland, S. *Nerves and Nerve Injuries*, 2nd ed. New York: Churchill Livingston, 1978, pp. 377–420.

462. Akil, H. Madden, J. Patrick, R. L., and Borchas, J. D. Stress-induced increases in endogenous opioid peptides: Concurrent analgesia and its partial reversal by naloxone. Kosterlits, H. W., ed. In *Opiates and Endogenous Opioid-Peptides*. Amsterdam: Elsevier, 1970, pp. 63–70.

463. Hayes, R. I., Bennett, G. J., and Mayer, D. J. Behavioral and physiological studies of non-narcotic analgesia in the rat elicited by certain environmental stimuli. *Brain Res.* 155:69, 1978.

464. Terman, G. W., et al. Intrinsic mechanisms of pain inhibition: activation by stress. *Science* 926:1970, 1986.

465. Axelrod, J., et al. Stress hormones, their interactions and regulations. *Science* 234:452, 1984.

466. Guillermin, R., et al. Beta endorphin and adrenocorticotropin are secreted concommitantly by the pituitary gland. *Science* 197:1807, 1977.

467. Lewis, J. W., Cannon, J. T., and Liebeskind, J. C. Opioid and non-opioid mechanisms of stress analgesia. *Science* 206:623, 1980.

468. Duncan, G. MJ., et al. Task-related responses of monkey medullary dorsal horn. *Neuros. J. Neurophysiol.* 57:289, 1987.

469. Hisey, J. A Search for the neurological mechanisms of ovulation. *Proc. Soc. Exp. Biol. Med.* 30:136, 1932.

470. Goldstein, A., Lowney, L. I., and Pal, B. K. Interaction of morphine in mouse brain. *Proc. Natl. Acad. Sci. U.S.A.* 68:1742–1749, 1971.

471. Wainapel, S. F. Reflex sympathetic dystrophy following traumatic myelopathy. *Pain* 18:345–349, 1984.

472. Joseph, R., Dhital, K., Adams, J., et al. Cluster headache: A new approach using fluorescent histochemistry of nerves in temple skin. In Rose, F. C. ed. *Migraine: Proceedings 5th International Migraine Symposium*, London, September 19–20, 1984. Basil: Karger, 1985, pp. 162–165.

473. Appenzeller, O. *The Autonomic Nervous System: An Introduction to Basic and Clinical Concents*, 4th ed. Amsterdam: Elsevier, 1990.

474. Appenzeller, O. *The Autonomic Nervous System: An Introduction to Basic and Clinical Concepts*, 4th rev. and Engl. ed. Amsterdam: Elsevier, 1990, pp. 27–30.

475. Appenzeller, O. *The Autonomic Nervous System: An Introduction to Basic and Clinical Conscepts*, 4th rev. and Engl. ed. Amsterdam: Elsevier, 1990, 157.

476. Basbaum, A. I. and Levine, J. D. Opiate analgesia. *N. Engl. J. Med.* 325:1168–1169, 1991.

476a. Raynaud, M. *De L' asphyxie locale et de la gangrene symetrique des extremites*. Paris: Rignoux, 1862.

477. Stein, C., Comisel, K., et al. Analgesic effect of intraaorticular morphine after arthroscopic knee surgery. *N. Eng. J. Med.* 325:1123–1126, 1991.

477a. Hilsted, J., Richier, E., Madsbad, S., et al. Metabolic and cardiovascular responses to epinephrine in diabetic autonomic neuropathy. *N. Engl. J. Med.* 317:421–426, 1987.

478. Seale, K. S. Reflex sympathetic dystrophy of the lower extremity. *Clin. Orthop. Related Res.* 243:80–85, 1989.

478a. Olsen, N., Petring, O. U., and Rossing, N. Exaggerated postural vasoconstrictor reflex in Raynaud's phenomenon. *Br. Med. J.* 294:1186–1188, 1987.

479. Basbaum, A. I. and Fields, H. L. Endogenous pain systems: brain stem spinal pathways and endorphin circuitry. *Annu. Rev. Neurosci.* 7:309–338, 1984.

479a. Hoffman, H. H. An analysis of the sympathetic trunk and rami in the cervical and upper thoracic regions in man. *Ann. Surg.* 145:94–103, 1957.

480. Comings, D. E. and Comings, B. G. A controlled family history study of Tourette's syndrome, II: Alcoholism, drug abuse, and obesity. *J. Clin. Psychiat.* 51(7):281–287, 1990.

481. Streissguth, A. P., Aase, J. M., et al. Fetal alcohol syndrome in adolescents and adults. *JAMA* 265(15)1961–1967, 1991.

482. Hokfelt, T. and Kellerth, J. O. Experimental immunohistochemical studies on the localization and distribution of substnace P in cat primary sensory neurons. *Brain Res.* 100:1975.

482a. Cooper, K. E., Johnson, R. H., and Spalding, J. M. K. Thermoregulatory reactions following intravenous pyrogen in a subject with complete transection of the cervical cord. *J. Physiol. (London)* 171, 1964.

483. Elfvin, L. G. Morphological studies on central and peripheral connections of sympathetic ganglion. Eranko et al., eds. In *Histochemistry and Cell Biology of Autonomic Neurons*. New York: Raven Press, 1980, pp. 335–340.

483a. Cooper, K. E. and Mc. K. Kerslake, D. Vasoconstriction in the hand during electrical stimulation of the lumbar sympathetic chain in man. *J. Physiol. (London)* 127:134–142, 1955.

484. Appenzeller, O. *The Autonomic Nervous System: An Introduction to Basic and Clinical Concepts*, 4th rev. and enlarged ed. Amsterdam: Elsevier Science Publishers, 1990, pp. 26–31.

485. Shearn, D. W. Operant conditioning of heart rate. *Science* 137:530–531, 1962.

486. Trowill, J. A. Instrumental conditioning of heart rate in the curarized rat. *J. Comp. Physiol. Psychol.* 63:7–11, 1967.

487. DiCara, L. V. and Miller, N. E. Conditioning of vasomotor responses in curarized rat learning to respond differentially in two ears. *Science* 159:1485–1486, 1968.

488. Patel, C. and North, W. R. S. Randomized controlled trial yoga and biofeedback in management of hypertension. *Lancet* 2:93–95, 1975.

489. Lang, R., Dehof, K., et al. Sympathetic activity and transendental mediation. *J. Neurol. Transmiss.* 44:117–135, 1979.

490. Greenspan, K., Lawrence, P. F., et al. The role of biofeedback and relaxation therapy in arterial occlusive disease. *J. Surg. Res.* 29:387–396, 1980.

491. Nathan, P. W. and Smith, M. C. The location of descending fibres to sympathetic preganglionic vasomotor and sudomotor neurons in man. *J. Neurol. Neurosurg. Psychiat.* 50:1253–1262, 1987.

492. Riosler, N., Reuner, C., et al. Cerebral spinal fluid levels of immunoreactive substance P and somatostatin in patients with M.S. and inflammatory CNS diseases. *Disc. Peptides J.* 11(1):181–183, 1990.

493. Finsterbush, A., Frankl, U., Mann, G., and Lowe, J. Reflex sympathetic dystrophy of the patellofemoral joint. *Orthoped. Rev.* 20(10):877–885, 1991.

494. Muller, A. and Farcot, J. M. Sympathetic nervous system, pain and epidural administration of morphine. *Agressologie* 32(5 Spec. No.):283–286, 1991.

495. Tountas, A. A. and Noguchi, A. Treatment of posttraumatic reflex sympathetic syndrome (RSDS) with intravenous blocks of a mixture of corticosteroid and lidocaine: A retrospective review of 17 consecutive cases. *J. Orthopaed. Trauma* 5(4):412–419, 1991.

496. Simon, D. Pain syndromes: case studies. *Iowa Medicine* 81(3):109–112, 1991.

497. Amadio, P. C., Mackinnon, S. E., Merrit, W. H., Brody, G. S., and Terzis, J. K. Reflex sympathetic dystrophy syndrome: Consensus report of an ad hoc committee of the American Association for Hand Surgery on the definition of reflex sympathetic dystrophy syndrome. *Plastic Reconstruct. Surg.* 87(2):371–375, 1991.

498. Levine, D. Z. Burning pain in an extremity. Breaking the destructive cycle of reflex sympathetic dystrophy. *Postgrad. Med.* 90(2):175–178, 183–185, 1991.

499. Bryan, A. S., Klenerman, L., and Bowsher, D. The diagnosis of reflex sympathetic dystrophy using an algometer. Royal Liverpool Hospital, England. *J. Bone Joint Surg.* (British Volume) 73(4):644–646, 1991.

500. Blumberg, H., Griesser, H. J., and Hornyak, M. Neurologic aspects of clinical manifestations, pathophysiology and therapy of reflex sympathetic dystrophy (causalgia, Sudek's disease). *Nervenartz.* 62(4):205–211, 1991.

501. Feldman, F. Thermography of the hand and wrist: practical applications. *Hand Clin.* 7(1):99–112, 1991.

502. Karstetter, K. W. and Sherman, R. A. Use of thermography for initial detection of early reflex sympathetic dystrophy. *J. Am. Podiat. Med. Assoc.* 81(4):198–205, 1991.

503. Bennett, G. J. and Ochoa, J. L. Thermographic observations on rats with experimental neuropathic pain. *Pain* 45(1):61–67, 1991.

504. Awerbuch, M. S. Thermography — its current diagnostic status in musculoskeletal medicine. *Med. J. Aust.* 154(7):441–444, 1991.

505. Irazuzta, J. E., Berde, C. B., and Sethna, N. F. Laser Doppler measurements of skin blood flow before, during, and after lumbar sympathetic blockade in children and young adults with reflex sympathetic dystrophy syndrome. *J. Clin. Monit.* 8(1):16–19, 1992.

506. Bej, M. D. and Schwartzman, R. J. Abnormalities of cutaneous blood flow regulation in patients with reflex sympathetic dystrophy as measured by laser Doppler fluxmetry. *Arch. Neurol.* 48(9):912–915, 1991.

507. McMahon, S. B. Mechanisms of sympathetic pain. *Br. Med. Bull.* 47(3):584–600, 1991.

508. Lofstrom, J. B. and Cousins, M. J. Sympathetic neural blockade of upper and lower extremity. In *Neural Blockade in Clinical Anesthesia and Management of Pain*, 2nd ed. Philadelphia: Lippincott, 1988, pp. 461–500.

509. Drummond, P. D., Finch, P. M., and Smythe, G. A. Reflex sympathetic dystrophy: the significance of differing plasma catecholamine concentrations in affected and unaffected limbs. *Brain* 114 (Pt 5):2025–2036, 1991.

510. Davis, K. D., Treede, R. D., Raja, S. N., Meyer, R. A., and Campbell, J. N. Topical application of clonidine relieves hyperalgesia in patients with sympathetically maintained pain. *Pain* 47(3):309–317, 1991.

511. Blockx, P. and Driessens, M. The use of 99Tcm-HSA dynamic vascular examination in the staging and therapy monitoring of reflex sympathetic dystrophy. *Nuclear Med. Commun.* 12(8):725–731, 1991.

512. Koch, E., Hofer, H. O., Sialer, G., Marincek, B., and von Schulthess, G. K. Failure of MR imaging to detect reflex sympathetic dystrophy of the extremities. *AJR: American Journal of Roentgenology* 156(1):113–115, 1991.

513. Schimmerl, S., Schurawitzki, H., Canigiani, G., Kramer, J., and Fialka, V. Sudeck's disease — MRT as a new diagnostic procedure [German]. *Rofo: Fortsch. Geb. Rontgenstrahl. Nuklearmed.* 154(6):601–604, 1991.

514. Feldman, F. Thermography of the hand and wrist: Practical applications. *Hand Clin.* 7(1):99–112, 1991.

515. Karstetter, K. W. and Sherman, R. A. Use of thermography for initial detection of early reflex sympathetic dystrophy. *J. Am. Podiat. Med. Assoc.* 81(4):198–205, 1991.

516. Bennet, G. J. and Ochoa, J. L. Thermographic observations on rats with experimental neuropathic pain. *Pain* 45(1):61–67, 1991.

517. Muñoz-Gomez, J., Collado, A., Gratacos, J., Campistol, J. M., Lomeña, F., Llena, J., and Andreu, J. Reflex sympathetic dystrophy syndrome of the lower limbs in renal transplant patients treated with cyclosporin A. *Arth. Rheum.* 34(5):625–630, 1991.

518. Merello, M. J., Nogues, M. A., Leiguarda, R. C., and Lopez Saubidet, C. Dystonia and reflex sympathetic dystrophy induced by ergotamine. *Move. Disord.* 6(3):263–264, 1991.

519. Ballard, E. M., Ellenberg, M., and Chodoroff, G. Reflex sympathetic syndrome secondary to L5 radiculopathy. *Arch. Phys. Med. Rehab.* 72(8):595–597, 1991.

520. Gillespie, L., Bray, R., Levin, N., and Delamartar, R. Lumbar nerve root compression and interstitial cystitis — response to decompressive surgery. *Br. J. Urol.* 68(4):361–364, 1991.

521. McNerney, J. E. Reflex sympathetic dystrophy. Traumatic and postoperative presentation and management in the lower extremity. *Clin. Podiat. Med. Surg.* 8(2):287–307, 1991.

522. Watson, H. K. and Fong, D. Dystrophy, recurrence, and salvage procedures in Dupuytren's contracture. *Hand Clin.* 7(4):745–755; discussion 757–758, 1991.

523. Kuschner, S. H., Brien, W. W., Johnson, D., and Gellman, H. Complications associated with carpel tunnel release. *Orthopaed. Rev.* 20(4):346–352, 1991.

524. Grundberg, A. B. and Reagan, D. S. Compression syndromes in reflex sympathetic dystrophy. *J. Hand Surg.* 16(4):731–736, 1991.

525. Schwarzer, A. C. and Schrieber, L. Rheumatic manifestations of neoplasia. *Curr. Opinion Rheumatol.* 3(1):145–154, 1991.

526. Blumberg, H., Griesser, H. J., and Hornyak, M. Distal post-traumatic edema — a symptom of a sympathetic reflex dystrophy (Sudeck's disease)? *Zeit. Orthopad. Grenzgeb.* 130(1):9–15,1992.

527. Webster, G. F., Schwartzman, R. J., Jacoby, R. A., Knobler, R. L., and Uitto, J. J. Reflex sympathetic dystrophy. Occurrence of inflammatory skin lesions in patients with stages II and III disease. *Arch. Dermatol.* 127(10):1541–1544, 1991.

528. Ammann, M., Hanggi, W., Schneider, H., and Hafelin, F. Sudeck's syndrome of the hip in pregnancy. A case report and review of the literature [German]. *Zentralb. Gynakol.* 113(15–16):895–898, 1991.

529. Wurnig, C. and Kotz, R. Algodystrophy in pregnancy [German]. *Zeit. Orthopad. Grenzgeb.* 129(2):146–150, 1991.

530. Uhthoff, H. K. and Sarkar, K. Shoulder pain and reflex dystrophy. *Curr. Opinion Rheumatol.* 3(2):240–246, 1991.

531. Wassef, M. R. Suprascapular nerve block. A new approach for the management of frozen shoulder. *Anaesthesia* 47(2):120–124, 1992.

532. Todd, D. P. Prolonged stellate block in treatment of reflex sympathetic dystrophy. *Agressologie* 32(5 Spec. No.):281–282, 1991.

533. Blumberg, H., Griesser, H. J., and Hornyak, M. Neurologic aspects of clinical manifestations, pathophysiology and therapy of reflex sympathetic dystrophy(causalgia, Sudeck's disease). *Nervenartz* 62(4):205–211, 1991.

534. Klein, D. S. and Klein, P. W. Low-volume ulnar nerve block within the axillary sheath for the treatment of reflex sympathetic dystrophy. *Can. J. Anaesth.* 38(6):764–766, 1991.

535. Arner, S. Intravenous phentolamine test: Diagnostic and prognostic use in reflex sympathetic dystrophy. *Pain* 46(1):17–22, 1991.

536. Varni, J. W. and Bernstein, B. H. Evaluation and management of pain in children with rheumatic diseases. *Rheum. Dis. Clin. NA* 17(4):985–1000, 1991.

537. Vanos, D. N., Ramamurthy, S., and Hoffman, J. Intravenous regional block using ketorolac: Preliminary results in the treatment of reflex sympathetic dystrophy. *Anesth. Anal.* 74(1):139–141, 1992.

538. Rumsfield, J. A. and West, D. P. Topical capsaicin in dermatologic and peripheral pain disorders. *DICP* 25(4):381–387, 1991.

539. Dore, F., Melis, G. C., Fumu, E., Casu, A. R., Vargiu, P., Azzena, M. D., and Madeddu, G. Role of densitometry and scintigraphy in post-traumatic algodystrophy of the arms. Initial diagnosis and monitoring during treatment with carbocalcitonin. [Italian]. *Radiol. Med.* 81(1–2):114–117, 1991.

540. Bickerstaff, D. R. and Kanis, J. A. The use of nasal calcitonin in the treatment of post-traumatic algodystrophy. *Br. J. Rheumatol.* 30(4):291–294, 1991.

541. Hannington-Kiff, J. G. Does failed natural opioid modulation in regional sympathetic ganglia cause reflex sympathetic dystrophy? *Lancet* 338(8775):1125–1127, 1991.

542. Olcott, C., IV, Eltherington, L. G., Wilcosky, B. R., Shoor, P. M., Zimmerman, J. J., and Fogarty, T. J. Reflex sympathetic dystrophy — the surgeon's role in management. *J. Vasc. Surg.* 14(4):488–92; discussion 492–495, 1991.

543. Coria F., et al. Episodic paroxysmal hemicrania responsive to calcium channel blockers. *J. Neurol. Neurosurg Psychiat.* 55:166, 1992.

544. Dore, F., Meliu, E., Casu, A. R., Vargiu, P., Azzena, M. D., and Madeddu, G. Role of densitometry and scintigraphy in post-traumatic algodystrophy of the arms. Initial diagnosis and monitoring during treatment with carbacalcitonin. [Italian]. *Radiol. Med.* 81(1–2):114–117, 1991.

545. Uhthoff, H. K. and Sarkar, K. Shoulder pain and reflex sympathetic dystrophy. *Curr. Opinion Rheumatol.* 3(2):240–246, 1991.

546. Todd, D. P. Prolonged stellate block in treatment of of refex sympathetic dystrophy. *Agressologie* 32(5 Spec. No.):281–282, 1991.

547. Feldman, F. Thermography of the hand and wrist; Practical applications. *Hand Clin.* 7(1):99–112, 1991.

548. Simon, D. Pain syndromes: Case studies. *Iowa Med.* 81(3):109–112, 1991.

549. Bower, B. D. and Jeavons, P. M. The effect of corticotrophin and prednisolone on infantile spasm with mental retardation. *Arch. Dis. Child.* 36:23–33, 1961.

550. Kato, Y. et al. *Proc. Soc. Exp. Biol. Med.* 158:431–436, 1978.

551. Bruni, J. et al. *Life Sci.* 21:461–466, 1988.

552. Mains, R. E. et al. Common precursor to corticotrophins and endorphins. *Proc. Natl. Acad. Sci.* 74 (3014B:3014 to 8), 1997.

553. Leao, A. A. P. Spreading depression of activity in cerebral cortex. *J. Neurophysiol.* 7:359, 1944.

554. Bourne, S. Treatment of cigarette smoking with short term high dosage corticotrophin therapy. *J. R. Soc. Med.* 78(8):64950, 1985.

555. West, R. Corticotrophin injections to treat cigarette withdrawal symptoms. *J. R. Soc. Med.* 78-12:1065–1066, 1985.

556. Cooper, J. R., Bloom, F. E., and Roth, R. H. *The Biochemical Basis of Neuropharmacology,* Oxford University Press, 1991, pp. 401–409.

557. Low, P. A., Opfer-Gehrking, T. L., and Kihara, M. *In vivo* studies on receptor pharmacology of the human endocrine sweat gland. *Clin. Auton. Res.* 2:29–34, 1992.

558. Stewart, J. D., Low, P. A., and Fealey, R. D. Small fiber peripheral neuropathy: diagnostic value of sweat tests and autonomic cardiovascular reflexes. *Muscle & Nerve* 15:661–665, 1992.

559. Low, P. A., Ed. *Clinical Anatomic Disorders: Evaluation and Management.* Boston: Little Brown and Co., 1992 (in press).

560. Sobotka, J. J. An evaluation of Afrodex in the management of male impotency: a double-blind crossover study. *Curr. Ther. Res.* 11:87–94, 1969.

561. Margolis, R., Prieto, P., Stein, L., and Chinn, S. Statistical summary of 10,000 male cases using Afrodex in treatment of impotence. *Curr. Ther. Res.* 13:616–622, 1971.

562. Morales, A., Surridge, D. H. C., Marshall, P. G., and Fenemore, J. Non-hormonal pharmacological treatment of organic impotence. *J. Urol.* 128:45–47, 1982.

563. Drew, G. M. Effects of alpha-adrenoceptor agonists and antagonists on pre- and post synaptically located alpha-adrenoceptors. *Eur. J. Pharmacol.* 36:313–320, 1976.

564. Brown, J., Doxey, J. C. and Handley, S. Effects of alpha adrenoceptor agonists and antagonists and of antidepressant drugs on pre- and postsynaptic alpha-adrenoceptors. *Eur. J. Pharmacol.* 67:33–40, 1980.

565. Guicheney, P. and Meyer, P. Binding of (3H)-prazosin and (3H)-dihydroergocryptine to rat cardiac alpha-adrenoceptors. *Br. J. Pharmacol.* 73:33–39, 1981.

566. Brown, M. J., Struthers, A. D., Burrin, J. M., DiSilvio, L., and Brown, D. C. The physiological and pharmacological role of presynaptic alpha and beta-adrenoceptors in man. *Br. J. Clin. Pharmacol.* 20:649–658, 1985.

567. Yamaguchi, H., Watanabe, S., Motokawa, K., and Ishizawa, Y. Intra-thecal morphine dose-response data for pain relief after cholecystectomy. *Anesthesia & Analgesia* (JC:4-8) 70(2):168–171, 1990.

568. Lipman, J. J. and Blumenkopf, B. Comparison of subjective and objective analgesic effects of intravenous and intrathecal morphine in chronic pain patients by heat beam dolorimetry. *Pain* (JC:opf) 39(3):249–256, 1989.

569. Steinstra, R. and Van Poorten, F. Immediate respiratory arrest after caudal epidural sufentanil. *Anesthesiology* (JC:4sq) 71(6):993–994, 1989.

570. Jacobson, L. and Chabal, C. Prolonged relief of acute post-amputation phantom limb pain with intrathecal fentanyl and epidural morphine.

571. Gourlay, G. K., Murphy, T. M., Plummer, J. L., Kowalski, S. R., Cherry, D. A., and Cousins, M. J. Pharmacokinetics of fentanyl in lumbar and cervical CSF following lumbar epidural and intravenous administration. *Pain* 38(3):253–259, 1989.

572. Baraka, A., Noueihid, R., Sibai, A. N., Baroody, M., Louis, F., and Hemady, K. Epidural meperidine for control of autonomic hyperreflexia in a quadriplegic undergoing cystoscopy. *Middle East J. Anesthesiol.* (JC: m9p) 10(2):185–188, 1989.

573. Ruch, T. C., Patton, H. D., Woodbury, J. W., and Toure, A. L. *Neurophysiology.* W.B. Saunders Co., Philadelphia, 1961, p. 363.

574. Trojaborg, W. and Plum, P. Treatment of "hypsarrhythmia" with ACTH. *Acta Paediatr.* 49:572–582, 1960.

575. Ochoa, J., et al. Chronic hyperalgesia and skin warming by sensitized C-nociceptors. *Brain* 112:621–6747, 1989.

576. Aminoff, M. J. et al. Dermatomal somatosensory evoked potentials in unilateral lumbosacral radiculopathy. *Ann. Neurol.* 17:171–176, 1985.

577. Mahoney, L. et al. Thermography and back pain. I. Thermography as a diagnostic aid in sciatica. *J. Am. Acad. Thermol.* 1:43–50, 1985.

578. Goodman, P. H., Murphy, M. G., and Sialtonen, G. L. Normal temperature asymmetry of the back and extremities by computer-assisted infrared imaging. *Thermology* 1:195–202, 1986.

579. Sherrington, C. S. Experiments in examination of the peripheral distribution of fibres of the posterior roots of some spinal nerves. *Phil. Trans. R. Soc. London, Ser. B* 190B:45–186, 1898.

580. Kerr, F. W. Structural relation of the trigeminal spinal in the cat. *Exp. Neurol.* 4:134–148, 1961.

581. Fredriksen, T. A., Wysocka-Bakowski, M. M., Bogucki, A., and Antonaci, I. Cervicogenic headache, Pupillometric findings. *Cephalalgia* 8:93–103, 1988.

Index

A

as reflex sympathetic dystrophy treatment, 7
Neuralgia
  postherpetic, 91, 92, 135, 149
  trigeminal, 69, see also TMJ disease
Neural pool overlap, see Sherrington's phenomenon
Neurodermatitis, 166
Neuroendocrinology, development of, 6
Neurokinin, in migraine headache, 76
Neurolytic block, 155
Neuroma, misdiagnosis, 113
Neuropathy
  diabetic, 91, 126, 147
    nerve blocks for, 151
    sympathectomy for, 157
  entrapment, 103
  toxic peripheral, 137
Neuropsychiatric disorders
  adrenocorticotropic hormone in, 140–143
  of reflex sympathetic dystrophy, 97
Neuropsychiatric tests, 163
Neurotensin, 42
Neurotransmitters, 117–119, see also specific
      neurotransmitters
  alcohol's interaction with, 97
  brain stem/limbic system content, 135
Nicardepene, 128
Nifedipine, 73, 128, 129
Nitrites, 73, 163
Nociceptive pain, 33, 49
  ascending relay system of, 30
  descending inhibiting system of, 30
Nociceptive system, 36–38, 58
No-let-go phenomenon, 100
Nonsteroidal analgesic drugs, osteoporosis and, 146
Norepinephrine
  antidepressant-related accumulation, 147
  brain stem content, 71
  convulsant action, 145, 145
  guanethidine interaction, 153
  in hyperthermic hot spot formation, 25
  muscle strength effects of, 152
  precursor, 132
  in seizure disorder, 144
  in spreading depression phenomenon, 77
  in stress-induced analgesia, 41, 42
  in sympathetically-mediated pain, 164–165
  sympathetic nervous system content, 30, 78
Norepinephrine spillover, 107

O

Ocean water, use in hydrotherapy, 126
Oligemia, 77, 78, 80
Oophorectomy, as cervical spondylosis risk factor,
      92
Operant conditioning, 150
Opiate receptors, in pain, 38
Opioid peptides
  endogenous, 38, 144, 168
  in stress-induced pain, 42
Opium addiction, 141

Orbeli phenomenon, 6, 152
Osteolysis, migratory, 96
Osteoporosis
  calcitonin therapy, 167
  estrogen replacement therapy, 146
  focal, 96, 167
  oophorectomy and, 92
  during pregnancy, 166
  reflex sympathetic dystrophy-related, 6, 8
  Sudek's, 126
Ovulation, 6
Oxazepam, 149
Oxygen, rogue, 73
  in hyperthermic hot spot formation, 25
  removal of, 126

P

Pain, see also specific types of pain
  localization of, 106
  objective versus subjective nature of, 110–111
  positive function of, 43, 44
  stress and, 40–41, see also Stress-induced pain
Pain history, 36
Pain measurement techniques, 105–106
Pain rating index, 106
Pain threshold
  in causalgia, 64–65
  cholecystokinin and, 70
  in complex chronic pain, 41
  in reflex sympathetic dystrophy, 97
  serotonin and, 73
Pain tolerance, cultural factors in, 9, 51–52
Paleencephalic pain, 51
Paleospinothalamic tract, 37, 49, 60, 74, 77, 79, 81
  modulators of, 51–56
Papaverine, 73
Papez circuit, 79
Paraplegia, 98
Paresis, 6
  sympathetic motor, 152
  sympathetic nerve block for, 151
Parkinson's disease, 95, 115
Pathologic pain, 44
Patient-controlled analgesia, 161
Pavlov, Ivan, 150
Periactin, 73
Peripheral arterial disease, occlusive, 102
Peripheral nerves
  electromyography of, 115
  in cephaptic reflex sympathetic dystrophy, 47, 48
  normal, 34
Peroxidation, 135
Phenethylamine, 73, 131, 132, 163
Phenoxybenzamine, 128–130, 163
Phentolamine, see Regitine test
Phenytoin, 149
Phobias, reflex sympathetic dystrophy-related, 3, 97
Physiotherapy, 113, 115, 125
  central biasing mechanism basis of, 69
  for cervical spondylosis, 93

Author Index